Preface

When I mentioned to my brother that I was about to finish this book, the first comment he made was something to the effect of, "What makes you an expert?!. You only have your own experiences to write about..." He was more or less right of course. However...

I have been a direct caregiver to four disabled or impaired people over the last twenty years. I have been a paid caregiver to one for most of that time, my wife became disabled fourteen years ago, her mother seventeen years ago, and my mother, now passed, about ten years ago. Now in truth, while I did no actual caregiving in-person to my own mother, I was involved in the process for that whole time, and had to at least deal with the family dynamics up until her death, and beyond now, three years ago. No, I am not an expert caregiver, but I came up through the ranks and have the scars to prove it.

This book is a compilation of what I and others have learned over that time, and how I managed, with help sometimes, to overcome some fairly insurmountable learning curves and still remain both relatively sane and relatively healthy. As you (the reader) will learn in the pages that follow, family caregiving is pretty much a lonely, unrewarding career, and definitely not for the faint of heart. It is also however, a vocation which can be personally rewarding and even funny sometimes, in amongst the wondering about how one ever ended up in such a place and how many others have ended up in almost exactly the same place, all with no idea on how it will all come out, save that the object of one's attention will in all probability one day pass on.

The first part of this book (or in hard copy, book 1) is composed of anecdotal advice, stories and tips on how one might survive certain issues which invariably arise in the caregiving of a family loved one. Mercifully for the reader perhaps, that section is only about 100 pages long.

The second part of this book (book 2) is a state by state (including Washington, DC and Puerto Rico) reference guide as to where a family caregiver might seek some assistance. It on the other hand is over four hundred pages long and personally verified as of the Fall of 2011. It can be obtained for at last look, free in the lending library on Kindle (Amazon.com), but is too prohibitively expensive to publish with part one.

Hopefully this book will be of use to its reader. If not, well there are others. It is not the end of my caregiving experiences to be sure, but at least it is a starting point/ reference book which with any luck the reader will find before he, she, or they are overwhelmed by the experience. My experiences are only broad representations which may or may not be remotely what you, the reader, will find caregiving to be. However, here and there I do provide some practical advice applicable to almost any caregiving situation, and that is perhaps the usefulness of my writings other than being an example of, "So you think you've got it bad...". In the event this book gets out there, then perhaps over time some readers might wish to share their experiences too, in which case I will update this book on occasion. Hopefully, one day even my own family members will do so, too (read the book for more).

Namaste solo traveler, and by all means, good luck.

I dedicate this book to both my wife for all her support

and to those unsung heroes out there who are currently

or have been family caregivers.

It is for you I wrote this one.

The

Caregiver's

Survival Guide

For Family Members

Dave Coe, and others ©2012 on Amazon Kindle

Revised 2015

Forward

"I know God won't give me anything I can't handle.

I just wish he didn't trust me so much…"

-So is reputed to be a comment from Mother Teresa, the patron saint in process of all care providers.

When I first began to write this book, I managed to get through about one hundred and fifty or so pages before I realized two important things. First, what I had written to that point was by no means the basically neutral foretelling of what it is like and what is necessary to survive as a care giver to a loved one. My words were full of anger, sarcasm and frustration from my more or less ten years of being a 24/7/365 caregiver, and that despite the best of my attempts thus far, I was writing a wholly negative book on the subject of care giving. In rewrites however, I have hopefully repaired these flaws (except my natural tendency for sarcasm). Humor is one way of getting through the tough spots, so please forgive me in advance if you find mine occasionally inappropriate…. And then get over it. I should also mention that in this final re-write, I began to update everything, but then decided that on the whole, it was better as an "over time" perspective than as history. What this book does additionally contain is another three years of caregiving experience for my wife, and also that of our seventy-one year old adopted son (I will explain that later). Needless to say, the never ending panoply of what might happen, what no one expected to happen, and "Oh God, what now"(s), does make their inclusions worthy of being added.

The second thing was that my teeth were rapidly deteriorating due to my inability to earn a sufficient income which would enable me to not only pay for my wife's medical needs but also the *at least* annual trip to the dentist. As I age, along with my loved ones, I am learning the truth of, the fact that if I as the caregiver am not in top form, how can I take care of anyone else. Being now over the age of consent by about forty years, besides not taking care of my choppers, I am getting arthritis, I have a constant pain in my leg due to a bike accident when I was a teen, and a variety of other things wrong with me which I basically have been unable to address. ObamaCare which has come since my last book is now the law of the land, but even that with its co-pays is not within my budgetary means, and if I can just hold out for a few more years until Medicare is available... I mention that here just to insert a tad of reality before you buy this book, to illustrate that no matter what, life and bills still happen. Being a caregiver to a loved one doesn't always pay those bills...

In any event, I do hope that you the reader will find some words of wisdom and perhaps even some solace in the chapters to follow. If not, well then go ahead and buy one of those namby-pamby goody two-shoe-er Pollyannaish books that most of the writers are hawking out there these days, it might make you feel better. (Like I said, I never could stop all my sarcasm....).

Test

1

Q: What do the following words have in common?

Anger

Frustration

Obligation

A: None are good reasons to make hasty or ill-advised decisions.

2

Q: What do the following words have in common?

Love

Friendship

Best Intentions

A: These aren't any better reasons to make hasty or ill-advised decisions.

Look, the truth of the matter is that when a person or family suddenly finds himself or herself or themselves in the situation of having a family member in need of live-in care, a great number of emotions are involved. Such is also true when you have been caring for your family member or friend for an extended period of time. Whether or not you are making the decision to be a caretaker or are engaged as an ongoing caretaker, many emotions do and will come into play, and you are therefore on notice to make no decision of any consequence on either the above groupings or any similar emotions. Positive and negative emotions tend to lead to mistakes, which are hard to undo, and in some cases, cannot be reversed.

For example:

You mom or dad who has been your bestest friend since the day you were born suddenly has a stroke and will be bedridden, probably for the rest of his or her life. What emotions come into play at that point? Well first, certainly you love that parent, which goes without saying. Second, he or she raised you, so tit for tat, right? And besides, he or she gave up everything so you could get those braces in six through eighth grade, and a certain sense of obligation would only be normal, if not a downright debt of familial honor. Put together, therefore, and with the best of intentions, you decide to move that parent into your home and make sure they have the kind of quality care that no stranger could ever possibly provide. Bravo for you.

Now, let's change the equation a little. You are married, have 2.2 children, a two income family, and barely see your two kids, let alone the "point two" one. You have a house, let's say, and it even has a spare bedroom for good old dad or mom to use. What are the consequences of this radical lifestyle change?

To begin with, you still have a mortgage on your home which has to be paid off, not to mention one or two car payments, the (#2) kid's orthodontist bills, and while number one child is about to go to college on a full scholarship, he or she still needs housing money and some sort of car to get around in. Because your parent is bedridden, you will have to quit your job in order to provide that one on one quality care you know you can give better than the local nursing home. Thankfully, that won't be much of a problem, at least for the first year or so, however, because you can sell your parent's house and use that money to replace your own lost salary. Phew, that at least is a relief. So, too, is the fact that your parent's Medicare takes care of the majority of the medical needs, they have a supplemental plan too, right?, and what isn't covered will at least be dealt with by his or her Social Security or retirement money, mostly... Okay, so financially, at any rate, it looks like a wash, at least for the next couple of years.

On the plus side, you gain all that quality time (see that chapter) with your infirm parent because you're now home 24/7. You can get back to family dinners not directly out of a box, there's all that reading you've been meaning to do in the spare time you know you will have, and then there's the volunteer work you've been meaning to put in down at the senior center or fish hatchery. When there is a plus side there is always a negative one, even if it remains at zero. But we shall cover that in another chapter. For now, let's change the parameters of our scenario a bit more.

This parent you are about to spend the next "X" number of years taking care of is in fact the one who just got out of prison after forty years of sentence for eating small child… Naw, that's a bit much. This parent is the same parent who was an alcoholic for the formative twenty of your now forty-five years, a mean drunk sometimes, and now suffers from dementia caused by that alcoholism. There were some good times along the way, but you moved out of the house when you were seventeen because of your issues, and it is only in the last few years that you have found some sort of common ground between you and your parent on which to form a familial bond, if only so the kids have grandparent and family history. You've overcome a lot to get where you are in life, but it wasn't easy in the beginning and you worked hard to rise above your early life. Oh, and you and your parent(s) live twelve hundred and thirty-six miles apart. Once again, married, 2.2 kids, house, cars, orthodontist and college. The truth of the matter is, this parent birthed and raised you, so you feel somewhat obliged to take over his or her care, considering.

On the plus side, home again 24/7, family dinners, reading, volunteering, and maybe after all that has passed, you can finally reconcile with your parent and make your shared few remaining years together be worthwhile. And perhaps you can…

In scenario number three, all is as in the first example, except you are single, live in a one -bedroom apartment, have a decent job and a functional, if not late model, car. Well, obviously you can't just give up your job, but selling your parent's house will allow you to get along for a few years. You could even move into his or her house, and because you were so thrifty as a child, you will have enough to get by on since you will not have to pay those bills which go along with being single. The plusses remain constant, and your love interest (if you have one), is even exceptionally understanding and willing to share your burden with you. Love, obligations and best intentions all come into play here.

Now I could go along making up all sorts of scenarios for the initial decision about why to become a familial caretaker, parent and child, child with two parents in need, spouse with spouse, etcetera; but hopefully you get the point. No matter whether your motivations for becoming a caregiver are all positive or across the board, there are things to take into account to which emotional rationalization sometimes blinds you. You have to take emotion out of such decisions as best you can in order to avoid some of the most common pitfalls such a decision will entail; otherwise you will have to face the consequences of your choices. Oh, and you might have noticed, "Anger and frustration" weren't used in the above examples. That's for two basic reasons. First, if you are angry at the prospect of becoming a caregiver, then probably you should avoid the whole matter entirely. If giving up your semi-annual trip to Hawaii is too painful for you to contemplate in order to be a 24/7365 caregiver, perhaps that is just the tip of the resentments yet to come. Secondly, anger and frustration tend to come about after the decision has been made, and dealing with their effects is a large part of a caregiver's life. In truth, half the purpose of this book is because of that fact, and hopefully by the time you are done reading it, you will be able to deal with your emotional reactions to, and in, your role as caregiver in a more positive manner.

Who This Book is For,

(Who it is not for...),

and a little about the author

With sufficient and extensive research, one can become knowledgeable on almost any subject. However, personal experience is about the only thing that will make one an expert when it comes to becoming or being a caregiver. I therefore have chosen to limit the scope of this book to that of the adult with familial adult type of care giving scenario, with apologies to parents who just found out that their brand new gift of a child is severely physically or mentally disabled, or both. While there may be aspects of this book that apply, I just do not have any experience with that situation and frankly, the worst thing I could do would be to fake it.

My experience comes from more than twenty years of personally being a caretaker to one or more adults, and incorporates the experiences of several others who have been so for a greater or lesser amount of time. I happened to be the primary raiser of my two wonderful daughters during their formative years, and that experience as a parent has helped me to deal with my current primary responsibilities as a care provider. I live in California where thankfully the state is wise enough to pay for in home supportive care of a loved one *(in certain circumstances...)*, I assume primarily since the costs associated with a nursing home are substantially higher. In my case I do not however receive any funds from the state for the care of my wife, but rather for our roommate who is at this writing seventy-one years of age and both mentally and physically disabled. In an odd twist of fate, it is that income which therefore prevents my wife from being at all eligible for assistance, and my wife's more recent disabilities which have now precluded me from obtaining any outside income to assist our standard of living. She and I used to share in the 24/7 of our roommate, but with the onset of her condition, I now am responsible for the care of both my wife and our roommate. Oh, and the state hasn't provided a cost of living adjustment for over three years, and in point of fact has decreased my hours somewhat in order to deal with its budget issues...

In our household, we therefore have both the situation of a disabled family member and of a disabled friend. Both require round the clock moderate to high level care, and both are more or less mentally competent. For the later of those two aspects, I am grateful. However, while she was fully fit, my wife and I also undertook the care of her mother for several years who was suffering from progressive dementia. That was our first real foray into the role (s) of being caregiver(s), and since then my own mother had succumb to that condition of being disabled. In that case it is my sister and then subsequently my brother who had to drastically alter her/his life in order to become a caregiver of a family member, and while their experiences are her/his own, there are many similarities of experience that we share. I also wish to note that I found the effect of my own mother becoming mentally disabled entirely different from that of my wife's mother and of taking care of our roommate. The artificial difference and one step back distance of her mother not being mine versus my own personal mother's condition was profound to me, and I will expound on that point frequently during this book.

The plain point of the matter is that no matter what any professional will tell you, if he or she has not taken care of a <u>loved one</u> personally, there is an experiential gap that professional can only begin to understand. When for instance one works in a nursing home, even if ol' Mrs. S. is the kindest, sweetest person in the world, the caregiver on duty gets to go home after eight hours and theoretically at least, have a life not related to care giving or to Mrs. S. Even a paid live-in care giver gets a night off once a week or so to do something unrelated to his or her calling. But for a family member who has chosen to be the one sole caregiver to another family member, well pretty much his or her or even their life will for the length of the illness or infirmity be primarily centered around the care of that person. No breaks, no, vacations, and no rest, unless there are others in the family who can provide a respite, at least once in a while, and we will discuss community assistance later). It takes a special person to undertake such a lifestyle, and excluding the future saints and those suffering from permanent Pollyanna-ness, it is for those people that this book was primarily written.

Care giving is a calling of sort. It requires commitment, the giving up of most or at least a great part of a private life, and it is usually long term. It has it's up sides, but statistically the experts tell us that there is not only a high burn out rate but also that the physical and mental health of the care giver, especially the solo care giver is often drastically affected for the worse by the time the need is no longer there. Abuse of the person being cared for is wide spread, and even in the best of circumstances, verbal fights occur frequently as a result of, if nothing more, normal personality clashes between the caregiver and the person being cared for. That is especially true of the adult child caring for a parent, as the reversal of parent-child roles is often hard for both parties to ever become comfortable with.

Now having stated a bunch of negatives, I do not mean to imply in any way that there are not positives to the care giving situation. Previously unheard of bonding especially is quite often a direct result of such situations, and particularly if there are children involved. Even in the case of dementia or other such memory loss disabilities and conditions where the short term memory is entirely or progressively non-existent, some of the aspects of familial history which suddenly come out of the parent's (et al) mind can make the experience highly rewarding for all.

A purpose of this book is to hopefully make the caregiving situation at least tolerable to all parties concerned. With luck, it might even make the situation pleasurable. The book is divided into a variety of chapters based upon what others and I have found to be important and have directly experienced. Some of it may help the reader, some of it may not, but all of it is based upon actual, front line experience in the trenches of being a caregiver for a family member or friend. What reference and assistance sources that can be found will be included along the way, and perhaps if it makes it to a second printing, there will be contributions added by some of its readers. At the end of this book, there is a state by state reference of all the available resources I could uncover for your referral and as a starting point in seeking help.

One more thing: When I was readying this book and the accompanying reference section for release I came to realize that some of the chapters were written so far apart that occasionally the timeline mentioned doesn't seem to fit in the general narrative. After some consideration, I decided not to fix the problem, rather determining that perhaps in showing the sometime differing viewpoints I have held over the nine years of writing this book (and now the revision) that I as well as everyone else can change with both time and experience, usually....

Dignity

As you meander through this book, you will eventually come across a chapter called, "I Can Do That Myself". The chapter deals with the general unwillingness of a once self-sufficient fully independent individual's pretty natural disinclination to give up all or most of the control of his or her life, even down to the petty insignificant details which in sum total can sometimes define us all. I decided after some review however, that it was important to insert comment right here upfront as to the true crux of that chapter, and the one overriding concept with which one should read and consider this book. See it up there, right in the middle of the page in sixteen point bold type? Yup; its dignity, a word which I have come to believe is essential for the preservation of the human spirit and the maintaining of some semblance of a positive forward looking lifestyle.

Dignity is an ethereal commodity which can never be given, but can always be taken away. It is a sense of self worth which can be respected from outside of one, or negated by the actions of others. And most definitely, it is something which only the individual him or herself can ever give up, and yet through the intercession of others, can be whittled away to nothing without much effort.

There are many clichés about dignity and its doppelganger, self worth. A man losing hope when he lost his job, a woman when the last chick left the roost (sometimes called empty nest syndrome), those are obvious examples. But how about something more basic like not remembering to buy that one item at the grocery store and coming home with everything except that one item, or perhaps just not being able to remember how to program the VCR? A person feels silly, a little embarrassed perhaps, and as one approaches and then passes fifty, begins to rationalize and even accept that such is a part of life. Such is a shared societal bit of life, and in a small way to be sure, also a minute loss of what…., that's right, dignity.

Now, imagine that you had a stroke or came down with some musculoskeletal wasting disease which prevented you from say, wiping your own bottom. How would that little loss of personal freedom make you feel, huh? Pretty s*$%tty, right? And then you have to go and ask someone else to clean that s*$% off for you! S*$% man, that's just out and out embarrassing! No one has had to do that since you were potty trained, and you even were the one to do it for the son or daughter you now have to ask to do it for you! Down goes your image of self worth, and down goes your dignity.

Alright, so maybe I was just a little graphic in the last paragraph, a little potty mouthed if you will, but someday, barring sudden death, you, me, and everyone you know will probably eventually have to ask for such forms of help from someone else. If they handle the situation in the best of ways, with a matter of fact *no big deal* style, yeah sure, your dignity might be slightly diminished, but you both will survive the activity. And if that activity is repeated over and over again with the minimum of fuss and agitation possible, then everybody comes out on top. It may not be win-win, but sometimes achieving neutral isn't the worst thing that can happen.

So, I guess all I am saying in the previous is this: As you progress through this book, and presumable your newfound or ongoing role as a caregiver, please remember to think of yourself once in a while in the role of the person you are taking care of. If something would mortify you, it will probably humiliate him or her. Loss of dignity is a soul killer, and it becomes <u>on day one</u> of your job to do your ever loving best not to do that to your charge. Griping about every last thing you do or being honey-tongued sweet (both of which are *very* degrading) is just going to make things worse for the both of you, as is denying your family member the right sometimes to just try… Obviously a person who has lost all muscle control on his or her left side shouldn't be allowed to try and drive a car. That would just be stupid. However, allowing and even encouraging him or her to learn to write with the non-traditional hand is harmless, and would not only give your charge a sense of accomplishment, but also an increase in personal dignity as well. The same goes for using the remote control or going off on some tangential project of which you personally do not see a positive outcome. Hey they get to try, right? I mean just like you…

Dignity, as I mentioned earlier, is ethereal. And without that delicate commodity of self worth, few can manage or survive. So, go on and read the rest of this book. Just remember that wither your *no longer competent or self sufficient one goest*, so someday probably *goest you…*

Emergency

Care giving is a life style that usually does not come with any sort of warning. While mental function loss is to be expected with an aging parent or friend, generally speaking the day it truly has to be dealt with is still unexpected and quite often even a shock. Such was the case with both my wife's mother and my own. They seemed to be functional quite adequately if at a diminished level due to their respective ages, and then all of a sudden one day, they weren't. The bridge clubs and lunches with friends were slowly dropping away, but there were reasons after all, old people get tired, they no longer had the interest in such things, stuff like that. But then you learned that their power had been turned off because they forgot to pay a bill, or they funnily enough got lost in the town they'd lived in for sixty years for the tenth time. Suddenly, right?

Often however, the decision to become and the need to have a caregiver for a loved one arise in an unexpected flash at 2:13 in the morning and some distance away. A heart attack occurs, or your dad fell down the stairs and broke his other hip two days earlier, and all of a sudden (again) there is a real emergency situation that needs addressing, and right then.

In my wife's case, the "sudden emergency" came upon both of us unexpectedly. She'd fallen on the stairs twice at work over a two year period, been out on disability and cleared for work twice, and then one day, *all of a sudden*, she found herself unable to drive her car. We had just moved into an apartment to make work closer for her, and having had a rather bizarre lapse of memory two weeks earlier which nearly caused her to forget where she was, she suddenly was unable to make her hands work properly. The former we, or at least I (more on this later) chalked up to perhaps her taking too many pain drugs for her aching back. But when the later happened, well we were by no means prepared. As it turned out, she needed two concurrent spinal operations immediately according to her surgeon due to some severe disk rupture issues, the higher of which was preventing her hands from functioning. The memory lapse might have been related. The point however is that in her case, while we knew there were problems, we were totally unprepared when they finally arose. We had some warning signs, but then again, who knew where they were going?

Sometimes, the emergency comes along in a slow, drawn out kind of scenario. With my mother in law, while we could see she was becoming somewhat more constrained in her life style due to her advancing age, she still seemed to have what we considered a life suitable to someone over seventy. She never had any complaints, and the first real inkling we had that there was something amiss was when we learned that some of her bills had gone unpaid and repeatedly. I'd only seen her a little bit more than on holidays as she and my wife were not exactly close, but when we started to pay real attention to her, the signs were definitely there. We moved her in with us three weeks later.

In my mother's case, there was what one might call a "through the cracks" type of scenario, but the result was still the same. She lived in Kentucky, and the three of us remaining kids lived out west. My dear sister-in-law as well as several friends kept visiting tabs on her, but… My sister-in-law's mother had suffered several major strokes years earlier, and my sister-in-law herself was for several months suffering from a rather unfortunate disease herself. Her visits to some extent tapered off as a result, and as my mom was a solitary person for the most part, her friends had been somewhat limited in their abilities to keep tabs on her. And to us three western living children, well she was generally happy and rarely forthcoming with her condition. It came to pass however, that one day her weekly cleaning woman came in and found blood splatter spewed from the kitchen to my mother's bedroom. She'd been fine the night before, but sometime during the night she had developed small blowouts and stomach (holes), which had caused her to start bleeding out her mouth and rectum. When the cleaning lady found her she was weak but alive, and due to blood loss we supposed, almost totally oblivious to the whole incident. To make a long story short, she was gotten to the hospital, the matter addressed, my sister the nurse flew there the same day, and things seemed to settle down and back to normal after a few weeks. Of course we were all worried, but as she seemed to be fine once more and the doctor concurred, well it was an unfortunate occurrence that simply required a bit more monitoring. After all, I already had two people to care for, my brother and sister had good jobs, and in my sister's case, she had children and grandchildren to be involved with. Crisis over, we all went back to the way things were, and a few months later it happened all over again. This time the doctor's looked a little harder, the holes were fixed, my sister stayed a little longer and even looked for work locally, and welllll, that time she'd barely gotten on the plane to go back home before mom started to bleed again. Once more, to make a long story short, the decision was made that mom needed an on the spot care giver and so my sister made the move.

There's more to that story as well as the others, and certainly the situations described are only faint examples of how people come to having to make the life altering decision about caring for a loved one. The similarity between them and so many others is however as mentioned, the sudden onset or emergency scenario which tends to cause the need. In my mother's case, while the bleeding has almost totally abated and was at best something sporadic from then on, that gave way either as a direct or indirect causative agent to her progressive dementia or memory loss. That caused my sister to make a permanent move to take care of her, and we can only be grateful that my mother's increasingly small world was at least for several years, a happy one. Such is as the reader will learn, not always the case and especially so when the loved one's mental faculties are fully intact. Even when they are not, the role reversal which transpires when a parent becomes a child's pseudo-child is an ongoing problem for both parties, and a large part of this book is devoted to just that issue.

In the next chapter, the assumption is that for better or worse, you have decided or been forcible thrust into the role of caretaker to a loved one. The latter would be for a variety of reasons assumed to be pretty much beyond your control, but in both cases, the need for a caregiver has become apparent, and the decision for you to take on the responsibility has been made.

Life Planning

(**Caution**: *This is a reality check chapter which is somewhat depressing and only poorly alludes to why with even the best of planning, you and your cared for one are now in the position you are in. It is only helped along a bit by sarcasm and bad humor and perhaps you should just skip past it and move onto the rest of the book.*) (*Thank you.*)

All right. So you've made the choice; the big unselfish commitment; the "Well, gee, isn't that what family (or friends) is/are supposed to do? No matter how well ahead you might have prepared for this day, no matter how much planning might have gone into your decision to become a caregiver, the actual reality of that is now upon you and it is time to deal with it. Of course if you never gave the matter a second though and all of a sudden in a fit of that emergency and your emotions you are now in charge of the well being of another, not to worry, there isn't that much difference between the two starting points. The reality of what you've chosen is about the same. However, before we deal with your side of the coin, let's spend a little time looking at how your loved one got into his or her need for a caregiver.

Now I was in a way, lucky, as were, in a way, my parents. Both their sets of parents passed more or less quickly, my paternal grandfather just after getting in a car at the end of a party, or in my father's case, after a mercifully short hospital stay. The latter, involving a second heart attack (ten years after the first) followed by three more while he was in the hospital. The pain of the moment for all grandparents and my dad was of course intense, but in all five cases, none required care taking at home for any real duration.

I can't speak to what may or may not have been decided and/or arranged by my grandparents in case of long term infirmities, but in my father's case, well he had everything well planned out; or so we thought. To begin with, Mom was supposed to go first. Not an unusual assumption by husbands of his generation, (although even then it was statistically improbable), but still an important point upon which he predicated all of his decisions at the time. Heck, he'd even arranged his pension in such a way that it was all paid out over fifteen years, a period of time which he supposed was sufficient for both mom to go first and for him to succumb to the family disease of heart attacks.

We owned a farm in upstate New York at the time, and planning ahead, he had uprooted mom and himself from the town in New Jersey in which they'd lived for some twenty years to a small section on the edge of the farm in order that my very responsible brother might keep an eye on them both in their declining and pre-planned non-lingering years. Oh, and just to wrap things up, he had even named an executer for his estate for after he'd gone, the local bank and its president, although unfortunately, he'd never told them about it. To make a long story short, my father's careful preconceived plan didn't quite work out.

To begin with, he went first, in the second half of his sixties. Having been golden hand-shook out of his job, this meant among other things that his fifteen year pension expired about nine years later with no one knowing that such an arrangement had been made. My mother had been the typical housewife given for their generation, she was a little younger than dad, she had almost no involvement in family financial matters, and to the best of my knowledge, had never even paid a utility bill in their thirty nine years of marriage. If it hadn't been for my brother and sister-in-law living a short quarter mile down the road, well it could have been an even harder learning curve for mom. At least that part of the plan went well, sort of…

Remember the executor my dad had named? Well because he and his bank had no idea of that naming, the farm was almost sold out from under my brother because my father had stipulated that my mother should have a decent return on her investment (dad had sunk more than half his savings and retirement into the farm), and that decent return was something farms just didn't tend to have. The bank was therefore legally obliged to sell the farm, and it was only after some expensive legal maneuverings that such was prevented. Now of course selling the farm had not been my father's real intent, but not knowing what my father truly wanted, the bank was legally bound to follow the fact of his will, rather than the intent. In the end it all worked out, but certainly not as my father had planned.

A few years later the farm was sold, returning an income to my mom in the form of some CDs, my brother and his family moved to the local town, and everything was more or less planned. They looked after her regularly, by phone if not in person almost daily, and all was right with the world, until one day the pension expired. Suddenly my mother's income was a quarter of what it had been, and her lifestyle changed dramatically. Still more or less healthy, she was able to keep her house (it was paid for), but the trips she'd been taking and the gifts of money she'd been bailing us kids out with for years had to end, and right then. My brother was now in his fifties, and unable to find a decent job in the area due to the gray ceiling, and together this caused the next

monumental change of moving both his family and mom down to
Kentucky, in order to be near my sister-in-laws parents and family. Not
the worst sort of thing to do actually; he still looked after our mother,
she had a nice condominium near a golf course, and as all of the condos
were owned by people her age, bridge groups abounded (golf and
bridge being her favorite pastimes). Mom pretty much had taken charge
of her finances by then, and in her mid-seventies, her situation was
pretty well where one might have hoped it would be.

And then my brother died. If it hadn't been for my sister-in-law rallying
together and taking over the oversight of my mom, well things could
have been worse. Of course there she was, taking care of her dead
husband's mother, her father had recently died her sister was sick and
her mother had one too many severe strokes which caused my sister-in
law to move her into her house… All of this was unforeseen by my
father's solo planning, my mom having been expected to go before he
did and all, but as mom was in relatively good health for a woman in
her mid-seventies and as our sister-in-law was the kind of person she
was, well things all worked out pretty well for a while. My sister-in-law
even got re-married, picking up a whole new set of familial ties, and if
it hadn't been for her husband's willingness to jointly take on the
responsibility of looking after my mother, who knows what we would
have done…

The final results were as stated previously, mom was of that writing
ninety years old, living in her own little world (a happy one, thank
heavens) due to her dementia, my sister moved there to take personal
care of her and in the process totally uprooted her own life, and if my
mother's family history is any judge, then she would be there for
several more years.

Now, why did I just tell you all of the above? Well to begin with in order to demonstrate the old saying, "something, something, something, planning, something, never goes as something, something, was planned in the end". The fact is there are lots of old sayings about planning and how it tends to go awry. I wrote the above narrative for two basic reasons. First, and more on this later, you will note that it wasn't until the very end that any of the three remaining siblings of my passed on brother had to be involved with my mother's care. It wasn't that we didn't love our mother or want to take care of her; it was just that things were going all right for her and we had our own lives to worry about. Oh sure, we three all visited from time to time, especially around holidays and on the way to someplace else, we all observed our mother slowly getting older, and most importantly of all, we all looked to mom as being the competent mother who had raised us since birth. It wasn't until that "emergency" described in the previous chapter that we had to rally and take action "all of a sudden", and since we are not nursing home type people, thankfully my sister was willing to drop everything and go to mom's rescue. My sister-in-law couldn't do it; she had enough of her own problems by then, and as for me and my older brother, well it would have been extremely problematic, to say the least. The one thing we did all four agree upon however was that as long as it was possible, mom should be allowed to live in her own house (familiar surroundings), and she needed 24/7 care. As I said, thankfully my sister was able to step in. But then again, she thought it was going to be for a much shorter period due to my mother's presenting illness. As with so many other things in this book, there will be more on that last point later.

The second reason I told you the previous story and perhaps the more important grounds to boot is for the simple fact that if you are not yet in the caregiver situation for your loved one, then you and he or she need to plan ahead now, and together. Let me state that again: Plan ahead <u>now</u> and <u>together</u>. No, you can't foresee everything that could conceivably come up, and no, if your loved one (and that includes yourself) is under sixty, then even talking about the subject is something which no one probably wants to do. Our life expectancies with all the new drugs and medical advances are now a good twenty years farther out than they were when we were born, so planning for catastrophic health issues should at least happen by age sixty, and earlier if there are ongoing health issues to be considered.

Now I wrote this secure in the knowledge that in my early fifties I will live a long time because: I do not eat the way my father did, and I am not nearly as sedentary as well, and despite the fact that I still smoke upwards towards two packs a day I simply can't die before my mid-seventies at least because I don't have any medical insurance. Phew, that was a sentence. Besides, with the coronary history in my family, and if necessary, I'll just let one of my two daughters totally alter one or both of their lives to take care of me. At least that's my rationale... Not!

Planning in my household consists of very little right now. My wife and I own little, so the whole estate issue is pretty much moot, she will be taken care of by Medicare and the state of California if I pass on first, and if I succumb to any serious illness, well hopefully I will die quickly because I sure as heck can't afford the debt load that would be incurred. Neither of us wants extraordinary measures used to prolong our lives, and if I do go first, then hopefully there won't be. *I just don't want to be a burden...*

Now there in that last sentence is perhaps the crux of it for most people, and the linchpin upon which most people base their planning and also delay asking for help when they need it from their family or friends until the problems are overwhelming. Let's now give a cheer for those in the first group; they at least tried to plan for all contingencies. Let there be no mistake about what is required for that to happen however, and that's lots of insurance and the money necessary to pay for it in preparation for a possible bad scenario. Americans are not known for their savings, which indirectly I suppose corresponds to why so few of us have catastrophic insurance, or even enough to carry us for our non-productive years of heavier and heavier medical and prescription usage. One good hospital stay these days can wipe out the savings of a lifetime even with decent insurance, and a couple, well prior planning may not lead to it but piss poor performance or reality may still result. Good insurance is getting more and more costly as what is covers is becoming increasingly less and less, and that's just the good news, for those who had it to begin with. For nearly half of Americans these days, including myself, insurance, or at least good insurance is just a fond desire. As savings don't exist and home ownership becomes increasingly harder to achieve even to be land poor, that half of Americans are wiped out immediately, owe more money than most of them will ever pay off, and as for that planning thing, well hopefully their/our benevolent government (federal, state, or local) will eat the debt and take care of us until our premature deaths due to the strain of it all… *Now at this point, Obamacare has just been legislatively instituted, and the effect is, well yet to be truly known, save there are a lot of people trying to remove every trace of what at best was merely a band aid universal medical plan. The parts I was most hoping for were getting some of my own medical insurance at a price I could afford, and fixing the non-competitive bidding with Medicare and Medicaid, both of which didn't make it into the final bill. Ahh me...*

So with or without prior planning, it just doesn't seem to be a pretty picture for the future. That ten or less percent of us you hear on the news holding ninety percent of the wealth will probably, and I emphasize probably will be okay. Our parents who managed to work for the same company for forty years, built a house, and put some aside might be able to weather the financial storm of catastrophic illness, at least for a while. And as for the rest of us, well as stated previously, hopefully we will die quickly, *so as not to be a burden.*

There's that word again, burden. Awful word that; and ninety-nine point nine percent of us would do a lot to avoid anyone ever calling us that, especially ourselves. I know one woman who in her fifties already plans to reside in a retirement home when the time comes; Another, a man who has the assets to pay for private care into his one hundred and fifties if necessary. Quite a few who know that their kids will look after them, and others, like me hope for a quick end. And a few who seem to have no difficulty "relying upon the kindness of strangers"… All have planned ahead in their own way, few planning successfully, most having no real clue as to what lies ahead, and all will probably not really be ready when the emergency comes. Inflation and other factors have taken their toll on even the most carefully thought out plans, and unfortunately, that messes things up.

At the time of the first writing, the Bush junior Medicare prescription plan had been implemented. For many it was a good deal, but for many others unfortunately, it requires the paying of a very large gap amount that will repeat on a yearly basis until they die. If those people basically live on their social security benefits, then that becomes a fairly hefty chunk of their rent and food budget. Or to put it another way, they don't have it. The fallout from this is still to be seen (as of this writing, see Obamacare), but it in its own way has a rather high potential for

qualifying as one of those emergencies which propel them into the care
by a loved one, even without being fully disabled.

All right, so what was the point of all of the previous in this chapter?
Well first, planning is a good thing, if you can afford it. Secondly,
there's an excellent chance it will only work somewhat, and third; well
this book is about caretakers and who they take care of, now isn't it....
It used to be true that if there was a family, that it went without saying
that come catastrophic illness and or disability, someone in that family
was expected without saying to become a caretaker, maybe even the
whole family. If a person was without family, if and when they became
unable to care for themselves, they went into a home, period. Post
WW2 however, things began to change. Family decentralization began
to occur regularly, thanks to interstate highways and suburbs. Group
residences not run by the church or privately came into their own, and
even the meanest son of a #%*^@ had some place to go other than
family. This is not to say that pre-WWII family members weren't
imposed upon or resented their being responsible for a parent or
whatever, but during the period from the end of the war through the
present, we all became used to the idea of independence and if you will,
ir-responsibility. We stopped thinking about having to be there for our
parents etal, and knew that as was true with our parents, our company
pensions, health plans, and careful savings would kept us going until we
succumb to death. Unfortunately, it didn't always work out for our
parents as planned, and as for those of us baby boomers and younger,
how many of us have expectations of ever receiving anything in the
way of a lifelong pension or have more than at best a few months or
rent or living expenses in the bank?

The truth of the matter is that while planning for a long retirement is
always a good idea, what perhaps is necessary now is at least planning

for the worst, too. Odds are you are going to live to be dependent on someone. Odds are you will live to have someone dependent on you if you do not already. Whether you are a burden or joy to have around, get used to those facts and read the rest of this book for how to cope in at least the latter case.

Heroes, Sidekicks,

And the Power of Invisibility

It goes without saying that at some point along your chosen path as a caregiver to your loved one, that someone is going to express something or another positive about your having done so. Now as mentioned, your loved one may occasionally in some ways resent you for your needed assistance, you might (and believe me will) even periodically come to the conclusion that you really screwed yourself up this time by making that emergency situation decision, but somewhere along your opted path someone will declare you a hero for what you are doing.

As a result of the above fact, you are going to have one of two reactions. First, you may very well choose to agree with the honorific. "Hell yes, I'm a hero! I gave up my nice comfortable freewheeling lifestyle to be constantly on call, never get a decent night's sleep, and fight regularly with my dad, mom, great aunt Gertrude just to get them to take a bath. Hell yes, I'm a hero!" Conversely, you may steadfastly and continuously refuse to accept even the slightest of thank you-s or praise for yourself sacrifice. "It had to be done, mom needs me, it's nothing special, no need for thanks…" You may even go so far as to get angry at people for simply suggesting you went above and beyond in making your choice to care for your loved one, throw it back in their face when they dare to say thank you and firmly stand on the self effacing principle that you were fortunate to have the honor of serving in a time of need.

In truth, there is also a third choice, a third reaction to where you now might find yourself, and the place where the majority of caregivers usually find themselves. It is someplace in the middle of the above two reactions. That place is the simple acceptance of being in the position you are in, and being the caregiver you find yourself to be. Sure, sometimes you are a hero, certainly there are enough people not in the position who either know they wouldn't want the job and admire you for your commitment, or who know they never could do what you're now doing. But for the most part, you are in your mind probably just *doing*, and that is the sum total of it for you, most of the time. You also sometimes will probably deeply and totally hate the position you are in, possibly even the person you are taking care of, and truly need someone out there to give you credit for your "sacrifices" (which because you feel so stupid for having made those sacrifices you will refuse to accept you made…). For the most part however, you just do what is necessary…

As mentioned early on, taking care of a loved one was for most of history just the way it was, and it is only with modern prosperity and the disbursement of families that care giving became something which someone else did for a loved one. This is not to say that there weren't still a lot of people who took on the personal role, but it is with the advent of insufficient insurance and greater longevity that more and more people are choosing or are forced to become a caregiver to a loved one. And such leads us into the area of sidekicks.

If you are lucky and have a large family with more or less strong bonds, your decision to become a caregiver probably came with the hero's usual companion and sometimes encumbrance, the sidekick. Perhaps your loved one has really good friends, or perhaps your spiritual or fraternal organizations have assistance plans for people in your situation; whatever. The point is that to a hero, a sidekick is an invaluable aide, and sometimes can preserve sanity, too. Being a 24/7 caregiver is if nothing else, a never-ending job. I liken it to my days as a farmer, where the cows needed to be milked twice a day (2-2-1/2 hours each, the barn cleaned (2 hours), cows fed and herded (1 hour). Now that added up to seven to eight hours, and did not include all the extra things that were necessary to operate a dairy farm such as the five months out of the years where one had to plant, care for, or harvest most of the cow's food (10-12 hours per day while it is going on), stringing fence, thawing out water pipes, etcetera. The point is however, that for much of the time, while a farmer is always a farmer, he may or may not always be working. Nonetheless, he is there 24/7/365. His day starts at 4:30 or 5:00 in the morning and doesn't end until after the last milking is complete and the last cow is fed, if then. Most farmers have families, and so the wife and kids also work despite their domestic or scholarly pursuits, and most farmers also have at least one relatively good hired hand on hand, too. Those family members and hired hands are the farmer's sidekicks, without which his farm would probably fail. Your sidekicks hopefully are those family members, friends, and social or religious affiliates who lend a hand when necessary. Make use of them. And no, things will never go as smoothly as when you alone are in sole charge of the care giving situation.

For those of you who have no "great" friends and family who can periodically jump in to help, there are other resources to be considered. No matter where you live, there is going to be some professional, semi-professional, or local through federal agency that can provide you with some sort of respite or help. Their help might and quite often does cost something, but sometimes, you just have to get away, ya know…. The only caveat to be aware of is this: Caregivers are quite often the lowest paid people out there, and while there are gems to be treasured among their numbers, you quite often get what you pay for these days. So be careful.

The third part of this chapter's title concerns the power of invisibility, and the longer you are in the role of caregiver, the more you will find you share that power in common with the one you are caring for. Disabled people are quite often invisible, and if you don't believe that, think about how many of them are out there that you never see. Like me, you probably always open a store's door when a disabled person shows up just outside. You may or may not wait to see if they can manage it themselves first (bootstrap Puritanism theory), but if they are having or it looks like they will have too much trouble opening that door, you bound over swing it wide, and accept their thank you for a charity well done. Now that's well and good, but how did that disabled person get downtown? What percentage of disabled people can get downtown for that matter? When a person becomes disabled, they become a statistic to all but a few select individuals, and even to those individuals, they lose much of their individual identity. With luck, they have a primary care doctor who recognizes them, maybe even a pharmacist and a few other support role people who know them well enough to call them by or at least recognize their name. Their friends slowly drop away, extended family tends to do so when there is no pending emergency going on, and so for the most part, you are your cared for person's main link to the world. Guess what? You are also unfortunately becoming invisible.

If as in my case, you have had to forgo the outside work place, then your world becomes pretty much the same one as that of your disabled loved one, with a few additions. I have personally made a great many casual acquaintances at the stores I frequent, and as far as social friends, why I know my wife's doctors almost as well as she does. My business contacts have pretty much slipped away, the extra-curricular activities we engaged in (friends) have dropped down to a minimum, and so I too am slowly becoming invisible. It's not all that different from what happens to many older people once they retire and their friends start dying off. The only difference is that I'm not old yet (at least by my standards)!

Personally I don't mind my invisibility all that much. I've always been pretty much of a loner, and once married, my outside activities basically centered around what my wife and I found mutually enjoyable. We still do many of them when she's up to it, and for the most part, the primary constraint we face is not her disability, and it is our diminished income's ability to fund a lot of those activities ($9.50+ per movie ticket plus snack costs, forget it). But if you really can't deal with an increased amount of anonymity in your life, then you are going to have to put forth the effort to prevent it. Sidekicks help a lot here, and so does knowing what you can and cannot trust your cared for person to do and not do. If he or she is having a good day, make use of it, damn it. If he or she is asleep and likely to remain so for an hour, go out for that walk and say howdy at least to the neighbors (potential sidekicks, btw). Providing that you don't belabor the issues or complain too much about your burden, they like so many will probably get around to calling you a hero at sometime during your conversation. Just let them…

A Personal Commitment

It goes without saying of course that a loved one who needs a caregiver will be committed to that life style. Well, actually it doesn't, but that will be addressed in short order. It does not go without saying however, that a caregiver is aware ahead of time of just exactly what he or she is getting into, or resultantly, how much of a personal commitment is involved in the decision to become a caregiver to a loved one. When my wife first became disabled, I didn't really think about the long term particularly. An operation or two, some convalescence time, and then I pretty much assumed that things would return to as they had been before she'd become infirmed. Oh sure, perhaps she might not have returned to full time work, even part time for that matter, but it was the height of the dotcom period, and well I could always make up for the income loss with the ridiculous salaries they were paying in those days. She, I assumed, on the other hand would recover sufficiently as to be able to at least keep house.

My sister as mentioned in a previous chapter, didn't have the warning I had with my wife as to the state of our mother's true health. She came for the crisis several times, left, and finally in a temporarily life altering change, moved to become the caregiver for our mother, for the few fulfilling and probably brief remaining months of mom's life. Well as things sometimes do, neither my sister nor I had any idea of how things would play out. We were clueless as to the realities of our respective situations, and as is true with so many caregivers of love ones, totally unaware of what we were getting into. Duh… (Inserted as an after the fact V-8® moment). My wife's situation has progressively gotten worse over the years, and my mother, well she was holding her own just fine until her passing, thanks to my sister's and brother's vigilance.

Care giving to a loved one is a full time occupation, and no matter if your loved one is a check in daily to make sure they've eaten well and not fallen overnight, or a turn every three hours, empty their catheter bag and try to keep them hydrated type, the overall commitment is emotionally at least, the same. You never stop worrying about your loved one's condition, you put many of your plans or desires on hold repeatedly and continuously for their benefit, and you have by accepting the job or privilege (as many will claim no matter how good or bad things really are), made a commitment with no definitive known end point or result, except possibly death. It would be perhaps nice if upon becoming a caregiver to a loved one, you could know in advance for instance that granny would without question pass on in exactly three months time, or sister Sally would recover satisfactorily from that car wreck to be self sufficient again in six; but life doesn't work that way. Granny may have had that first major debilitating stroke ten years ago, the dementia has progressed the last five, and she's been bed ridden the last two. Sally was getting better for a while before that third operation but since then can't even walk anymore, let alone be self-sufficient. Or maybe in Sally's case at least, she recovered in four months instead of six. You just never know what is going to happen over time, and that's where the commitment part puts on its main weight.

The first inclination of a caregiver when assuming their new role is to plan. They plan for the supposedly known (well the doctor says she has only a few months to live), they plan for the certain (I'll have breakfast ready at eight am, bathe him at eight-seventeen, make the bed at eight-thirty), and plan for themselves (I'll use my accrued vacation time to get over the initial period, and surely be back at work within the allowed time in order that my vested retirement rights don't disappear) (oh, and I will definitely go the movies at least once a week and finish that novel [quilt, ship model, graduate degree, whatever) I've been putting off.

Well frankly, doctors play the actuarial odds (they guess a lot based on experience), organization falls down in the best of circumstances (combative patients may not want a bath… for weeks), and your personal goals take a backseat to the needs of your loved one, almost constantly (you're going to get tired). The tendency to micromanage or simply the desire to plan everything out ahead of time is useful in a business relationship, but the plain facts of the matter are that if you cannot live without organization in your life, you will probably have a bad time being a caregiver. Some things in a care giving situation can be planned out, something have to be, and in the case of both, the caregiver is going to have to adjust most of the time to the day to day changes that are sure to occur.

For example: How many diabetics are actually religious in their testing and insulin taking needs? How many of them <u>never</u> eat outside their diets or do something which will in some way alter the way their body requires insulin. A diabetic is a self-actualizing caregiver to his or herself, and even they (or 99.9% of them) can't plan out everything or every contingency with perfection; and they're doing it for themselves! So how can you as a caregiver hope to plan your care giving life out any better?

I said in the opening paragraph that a loved one who needs a caregiver will or should be committed to that life style. Well, maybe. Being totally dependent on another person is for most people a really hard position to be in. Put yourself in that situation for a moment. Suppose just to get a drink of water you had to ask someone else to get it for you. You can heft the glass yourself. You can even get rid of the results yourself later on (void, pee, piss). The only problem you have is that since you are currently wheel chair bound and the counters are not low enough, you cannot reach any faucet in order to get the water into the glass your caregiver has thoughtfully placed out for you (abrogating the need to actually reach one down from the cabinets which are even higher than the sink and counters). Your caregiver even put out a pitcher of water for your consumption that morning, but as you drank it all earlier, you now need to get help just to quench your thirst. Now, let's suppose that you have to ask someone else to get you a glass of water ten times a day. If you don't you're going to get really thirsty after a while. Now go one step further and imagine you have needed that help and just that help for six months, a year, ten years. How would that make you feel about being a person? You might even grow to resent your caregiver because they can get that glass of water and you can't. Sounds ridiculous, right? I mean that caregiver, your attentive wife, your loving daughter; your grandson (and his family) is/are only tying to help. That person is only there to continue your ability to have a glass of water. And you, because you can't get that water yourself are resentful of their being there and conjointly, your inability to get that glass of water your own darned self! But it happens…

Let's look at say a situation like this: Your father, paragon of strength and self-sufficiency; Eagle Scout at ten, Medal of Honor recipient, founder and CEO of Amalgamated Expensive Stuff, and the one who always could do and fixed everything that was wrong for everyone in the family, well he has begun to suffer from Alzheimer's. What's perhaps worse, well he got lost driving home from work a few times last month; the same work he's been driving home from for thirty years. Now, he still knows who you are, your kids names and who the President is, but his memory is definitely slipping, and it has led to his eventual loss of a driver's license. What we are talking about here therefore is a totally self sufficient man who is now due to his illness just to the left of being able to properly care for himself. What we are also talking about therefore is a man who is at least periodically going to resent the hell out of being "cared for", at least periodically and frequently enough to make your task difficult at best and downright unpleasant at worst.

To understand the above scenario better, first look it at from his point of view. He spent his life being the "go to" guy for whom no task was too daunting and almost everything was possible. Suddenly, he has to rely on someone else, in this case one of his children to whom he was such a paragon, to do so many of the things he, as we all do, took for granted. He, because of no physical disability, now needs someone to do for him instead of being the do-er, and the help he needs (in this scenario) isn't even for big things. It's for remembering to take his meds and being driven to the doctor and barber and what was the name of his favorite cousin… And he feels both helpless and that you are treating him like a child! He's your father for pity sakes!

All right, let's do one more. Your son of thirty years just mated with a tree hot dogging it down the ski slopes. His spine is messed up totally, he is now disabled for life just for a moment of pleasurable bravado that effectively ruined his whole life, and he is in constant pain. Now this son of yours was, excepting for being a slightly rebellious teenager was always a good boy, polite to his elders, a good student, and generally an agreeable cuss. Forgetting for a moment his disabilities and all that will go with that for the rest of his life, he is now in constant pain as mentioned, and despite a really good dose of pain pills, muscle relaxants and anti-depressants (he had good catastrophic insurance), you have begun to learn that a) all those pills quite often don't really deaden the pain, and b) he is getting more and more irritable as time goes by as a result.

Did you ever pull a muscle in your back? Do you remember snapping at people as the days wore on and the pain just didn't seem to go away? Now think about making that pain something which you've been enduring for oh, three years and which the only relief from is by virtually making yourself unconscious and your insurance will only fill "x" number of pills per month and you are already a few days ahead of your needs and you're going to run out before your next refill, and, and… Your backache went away, eventually. What if it never did? How would you treat people after having it for a month, a year, five years? Oh, and just as a side note, medications for the most part have side effects. With many muscle relaxants and pain pills it is constipation; really bad and continuous constipation. And guess what? All that intestinal pushing leads to among other things, more pain.

Now in the above scenarios, your son doesn't mean to constantly snap at you, your dad doesn't plan to be constantly disagreeable, and as for yourself being in a foul mood because you always have to ask for that glass of water, well you are of course really grateful for the help and how could your care giver possibly think you are mad about being cared for? Being beholding to another, especially for dumb reasons (to the dependant at least) is not a state of affairs to which we humans adjust easily. Early on in my second marriage, I remember lashing out at my wife when while I was recovering from some minor surgery, she had not gone to the effort to find a milk shake with my fast food dinner when their machine was down, whilst if positions had been reversed, I would have gone to at least one other such establishment in an attempt to procure the desired milkshake. Normally, I would have let the matter drop. But I was hurting, slightly doped up, and feeling generally disagreeable at the time and so I lashed out at her for her lack of consideration. And why? Because I couldn't make the trip out and do what I would have normally done and it isn't a good excuse but that's what I did and felt. I didn't like being helpless and I attacked the nearest convenient target, my wife the caregiver. Now admit it, you've done the same thing at least once in your life for some sort of similar reason. I mean nobody is that perfect. And I suspect you even felt really bad about what you did sometime after the fact. So imagine living your life under that sort of pain all the time and think about how you would really act as a result. Now think about being the caregiver to that person…

The commitment to becoming a caregiver comes in a variety of levels, from being there if needed, to being there constantly. It can be a pleasant experience under the right circumstances or it can be a commitment that eventually robs you the caregiver of your health, your identity, and pretty much everything else you once thought important. Sure you get a gold star for being the one who stepped forward, but even Mother Teresa is quoted, as saying she often really hated her chosen job. It was simple that it needed to be done and no one else was there to do it. Your commitment is one of your own choices, presumably, and how and to what degree it affects the rest of your life is the question you will have to find an answer to along the way. The choice is yours, and hopefully, throughout the remainder of this book you will find suggestions that will help you remain a healthy and reasonably happy individual while you take on the responsibility of the care for your loved one. Some of those suggestions concern ways to manage to at least a certain degree the needs of your loved one. Some will concern ways for you to stay sane and healthy. And some, well you will have to decide in the end whether or not they apply to your situation at all. The two I will however suggest right now before you even read the rest of the book are I believe the two you will find the most useful and necessary for your survival overall. To wit:

Keep thine sense of humor,

And

Forsake it thee the taking of it personally.

You won't be able to follow either of these suggestions every time or all the time, but both will go a long way to keeping things in perspective. Oh, and of course the suggestion made in the opening about not making permanent decisions in an overly emotional state (like that will ever happen…).

I Can Do That Myself

(Damn It!)

We touched in the previous chapter on the subject of being dependent on another and what it can do to one's self esteem. The idea of being self-sufficient one day and then becoming suddenly unable to do for oneself to a greater or lesser degree is anathema to most people. It just isn't the way nature or the bootstrap protestant work ethic philosophy under which most of us were reared intended us to be, if you will. In the wild (and in our distant past), when the vibrant young hunter becomes disabled or too old to provide for his or herself, what happens? Well they slowly starved to death and hopefully didn't get eaten upon before they did. Man on the other hand has chosen to endeavor to prolong life as long as possible, and if not one's own, then that of others around us. Modern medicine, better diet, familial and social dynamics, and the fact that there are no predators bigger than us waiting just outside to attack our fallen bodies, have all come together to create the uniquely human sub groups of care giver and care receiver. Oh sure, the queen bee is attended by her thousand of drones and like that, but if she falters, whallah! She's ousted by a younger healthier replacement and the hive goes on. Man has made the conscious choice to tend to his fellow man, and in the case of a loved one being cared for; man has further chosen to go the extra mile. Such is not always to the pleasure of the loved one, however.

For the fully, or mostly so, in-tact mentally disabled, being "cared for" is quite often a very painful and double edged sword. On the one hand they need the care, for whatever reason and to whatever level, but on the other, that care can slowly erode the last glimmer of self-respect the person being cared for has left, and that can and quite often does lead to some serious problems for all parties concerned. While the physical work may be harder, that is why a nice comatose person <u>could</u> be almost considered an easier loved one to care for. At least they don't feel dehumanized and can't take out their pain on their caregiver.

As of this writing, my wife is currently going through not only the loss of mobility her condition had brought about, but also a constant high level of pain her medications don't quite often begin to abate, **and** menopause, all at the same time. Her memory is shot, the goals she sets for herself one day are gone the next, and despite the best of intentions on both our parts, we are frequently on the brink of a fight these days if not in one. Heck, if we don't talk about divorce at least once a month we're particularly lucky, although so far at least, no one has wanted to take matters that far yet. It isn't that we don't still love each other, but with all the resentments that build up <u>on both sides,</u> sometimes I don't know how we manage to hold things together. (Now this was one of those early sections I mentioned at the beginning of the book where what was has changed and what is <u>is</u> fundamentally different. I mean she is no longer in menopause, which has helped considerably. I am much more pliable, and she isn't as touchy. It works for us, mostly).

My wife's big issue is the one under discussion in this chapter, that is to say her hating to be dependent on me for almost everything, and the resultant loss of self esteem and resultant guilt she feels from being in that position. Mine is primarily my failure to "fix" her, the failure of my attempts to successfully deal with her self esteem issues quite often, and my resultant guilt for not being able to therefore successfully meet her stated and unstated needs accordingly. Are you beginning to see a pattern emerge here?

Let us revisit the example in the last chapter of simply getting a glass of water. The sheer frustration of not being able to do so oneself has to be terribly demoralizing after a while. Now add to that the loss of being able to drive oneself, and sprinkle in a little of "I really wanted codfish chips for breakfast and you forgot to buy them", and it must get overwhelming sometimes for the person being cared for. Now to be sure, if his or her primary disability is one of diminished mental capacity, then the issues tend to be from the past, but even that eighty year old father of yours who has advanced Alzheimer's drove for seventy-five of those years, and sometimes he just plain misses that freedom. No, he can't remember your name sometimes, but yes, he still wants to hit that open road from time to time nonetheless, even if he doesn't know where that road is anymore. It's just the way he and we are.

So what do you do? Frankly, sometimes, you have to let them try. Now I'm not saying that your aging father with Alzheimer's should be allowed to drive, but I am saying that with proper precautions, he should be allowed to do whatever he still can safely.

For instance: My wife has some friends a few towns away by mass transit. Sometimes, and initially against my better judgment, I've simply had to let her go visit them, and by herself. Now her wheelchair has about a five hour life on its battery. The transit system is about forty-five minutes away on our end, and thirty from her friends. Added together that makes two and one half hours of usage, and that leaves about the same for other purposes. If everything goes according to plan and it doesn't rain and short out her wheelchair, she should be able to have a grand time and I need to keep my worries down to a minimum, for her sake. No, things don't go smoothly every time, and yes, I have had to rescue her and her chair more than once. But you know what, she had fun being in control of her life again if only for a little while. And that "fun" is what makes her life bearable, sometimes.

Now I am not advocating letting your mentally impaired father drive the car, by any means. But perhaps he can if physically able be allowed to use the riding mower sometimes. Perhaps, even if he won't remember it five minutes after the fact, he should be allowed to go play miniature golf with you and your friends. Why not? You're there. He won't get lost.

Self-actualization is something which even our pets seem to enjoy, so why not our diminished capacities loved ones? If Spot derives great pleasure from playing fetch, why shouldn't mom equally enjoy the needlepoint that she so loved to do before she forgot where she left the materials (and so what if she ends up with a twenty-eight foot arm on the sweater she's knitting, she is enjoying the effort). Those were examples of people who are mentally not always with us. My wife has a friend who is a full one hundred percent quadriplegic. He can't do anything for himself except use his mind and his head. But he loves poker and he loves to create art. Now he can't hold cards or a paintbrush, but he can tell his caregiver what cards to hold, and he can through a breath operated device paint via his computer, and that makes him feel almost human again. So where's the harm? He now even has a website up for selling his art and the art of other disabled people. Not bad, huh?

A caregiver's instinct is to do one of two things; to do everything and to do as little as possible thereby forcing the person being cared for to do something. Unfortunately, both ends of that spectrum of all or nothing can be the wrong things to do. Your loved one probably won't appreciate your over zealousness, and you probably will resent having to do everything or their inability or lack of interest in doing what you want them to do. It becomes a lose-lose situation. And no, I am not talking about the extremely rare situation where a person being cared for **chooses** to be totally dependent. Such examples are rare in my experience and probably need outside help if that's the case. However, for those who simply want to do, something, anything, your encouragement and help with that can be invaluable in that regard. It's like the Desiderata said, knowing when you can help and when you can't.

On the other hand…

As sort of post script to this chapter, there is one occasional and very frustrating, infuriating, and totally unreasonable word which your love one may bring to the table. That word is the definitive "No", and no matter how it is said, sometimes it will be insurmountable.

As stated previously above, it is part of your job (while your stomach muscles clench up) to encourage and even cajole your loved one to do the most he or she is capable of doing. Hopefully you will be successful in such endeavors. However, what about those situations which by their very nature are really bad ideas and ones which you simply are unable to prevent? I'm talking about those situations where your disabled loved one, for whatever personal reason, does not choose to go along with your better judgment on a given matter, and you are, for whatever reason, totally unable to do anything about it.

By way of an example: My wife goes through patches where she sleeps the day through, getting up around dinner time or so. She has in that process missed the correct timing on her meds, at least one meal, and in general screwed up her own day, if not mine. Five or six hours later, I'm ready to go to bed (changing my hours to coincide with hers has proven over the long haul and several years of experience not to be the answer), and she is not. She has taken most of her now condensed (in timing) meds, is a little groggy from them, and I am exhausted. Since she is a smoker I know the situation is unsafe, but quite simply, she refuses to go to bed (which might change her schedule back to coincide more closely with mine). What can I do?

In the end, sometimes you can only do your best, frankly, and then trust to God to look out for all concerned. Extracting promises, providing safeguards, and even threatening (such as "if you drop one more cigarette I will not allow you to smoke") only goes so far, and eventually, your loved one simply wins out. If you are the only caregiver you simply cannot be on guard against all eventualities twenty-four hours a day, you can only do your best. I strive to prepare for the worst case scenarios, and hope for the best outcome.

Now I did not add this section in order to depress you. Most of the time your care will be sufficient, and probably even more so than say the 1-40 staff to patient night ratio in a nursing home alternative that is the only other clear out. In that *inevitable* end you can only do so much, and for your own sanity, you had better learn to be copasetic about it. In nearly 16 years of being my wife's caregiver I haven't lost her yet (or the roommate for that matter [21 years]), so……….. I do win the majority of the time after all, if only because she knows that I'm looking out for her. And when I occasionally don't: Well I trust in God's Diving Intervention, and know simply that she's a butthead sometimes.

Personal Space

Do you know what the most popular kid in school and the majority of celebrities have in common? Here's a hint: If you've been a caregiver for any length of time, you have it in common, too. Personal space is a commodity so precious to most people that it is one reason we are ruining our environment. What, you say… Yup, according to recent surveys, the primary reason that most people own a car after convenience is… you got it; personal space. Despite many fine mass transit systems in existence today, and the cause of so many others having long since gone into demise is our overwhelming desire to have, if even only for a few brief moments, some personal space. It is why for instance, when for perhaps ten more minutes a given person might be able to save ten to twenty dollars per day by using mass transit, he or she still insists on taking the car, and by his or herself. It is why dads have garages and basements, and moms have garages (I'm being politically correct here) and sewing rooms. It is sometimes simply a place to blissfully be alone for a few minutes; to hide, if you will.

Caregivers and their loved ones live in a world where personal space and its close cousin, alone time, are at a premium, and resultantly they like everyone else tend to get on each other's nerves after a while. Unfortunately however, that can and often does lead to problems, and sometimes worse. Because of my wife's and our roommate's need for care and supervision, it is a rare occasion indeed that takes me out of the house for more than a few hours per week. Heck, before the increase in gas prices, I would find almost any excuse to go out by myself for at least a quick errand nearly every day. It is also why I so cherish it when she and the roommate are both napping in the middle of the day and I have no pressing chores. For perhaps an hour or two, I can just not be on call, not do anything of consequence, and not be waiting for the next request (remember the glass of water?).

Now my wife understands my need for some personal space and alone time because she needs and wants it too. The major difference between us, however, is that I can at a whim just hop in the car or go out to the common garden at our apartment complex, and she for all the obvious reasons, can't. It takes a good day for her to even have the freedom of pain and the mobility to want to go outside, and for her, even when those two conditions are met, the to heck with it knowledge that riding (bumping) around in her wheelchair is going to give her more pain (try going over a speed bump in a wheelchair. It can be jarring). Her usual solution is to take a nap, which conversely gives me some alone time at the same time. Our housemate on the other hand pretty much chooses to stay in her room, which makes her presence not a real factor in this discussion. The one comment I will make however is that my wife and I both cherish the rare occasion that our housemate goes out for an extended doctor's visit or wheelchair jaunt. Sometimes just having one less person in the same apartment is an increase in personal space for us as a couple.

Hoping For a Draw at the End of the Day

(Tomorrow Will Be Better)

As of this writing, (This part was written almost ten years before the rewrite), (who knows when you will read it), my siblings and I are engaged in a rather unfortunate battle about well, nothing. The battle concerns my mother; the parties in apparent opposition are my sister (the caregiver), my brother, sister-in-law, and myself. The weapons of choice are feelings, mood, economics, and of course familial guilt, and the battlefield comprises the internet and the telephone line. And quite frankly, I haven't a clue what it is all about.

Well that's not exactly true. I have endeavored to explain how the decision was made for my sister to become my mother's caretaker, and what she had to give up in order to do so. I believe I have also made reference to her having forbidden us to make any fuss over her for having been the one to give up so much for an undetermined amount of time. I know from personal experience where she is coming from on that point, and while the exact parameters of our respective care giving situations differ, the basic underlying truth they both share is the same. Neither of us wants to be doing what we are doing, both of us made the decision to do the job none-the-less, and both of us feel guilty for not loving the job and therefore what the heck is there to praise.... The major difference between us is however that she is extremely unhappy in her role, getting more and more depressed as it continues and she misses out on what's happening "back home". Me, I accept my fate for the most part, and I am home.

Now this seems like as good a time as any to bring up the topic of family dynamics, both prior to the care giving experience and ongoing. While I will get into the meat of that issue in a moment, if I were going to sum it all up ahead of time, I would say the following:

> If the family members involved in a care giving situation (or any other for that matter) have all matured into adulthood, lived life as adults, and become pretty much set in their respective ways, then it is likely that they are going to behave in those self-same behavioral patterns once a care giving situation arises.

In other words, there comes a point in all of our lives where we are who we are, and that is unlikely to change just because the game changes. Type "A"s will remain type "A"s, loner's will remain loners, and your brother or sister who can irritate the heck out you with a few carefully tossed words, is still going to irritate the heck out of you with a few carefully selected words, care giving situation or not. The difference now being that that brother or sister or aunt or uncle is now the caregiver to your family member, and therefore not only the one in the day to day trenches, but the one who is basically in charge of the care giving situation. Given the best of all scenarios, there will be issues that arise, but when problems do develop, as they always will, especially with the caregiver, and then the question is what to do next.

All four of the original siblings in my family are or were at least fiercely independent. So much so, as a matter of fact, that sometimes we would do things in direct opposition to common sense simply in order to prove our individual independence (or at least I did, and occasionally still do. My two remaining siblings will have to accept or deny the rap in their own conscience, regardless of what I think to be true in their respective cases). As to my sister-in-law, she has always struck me as a feisty follower, or someone who prefers others to lead, but will upon occasion fight tooth and nail as regards something she feels strongly about. What this has all meant over the years is that on a rare (hah!) occasion, we have jointly and severally been known to get into tiffs. No broken bottles, no pistols at ten paces, but as we are all extremely good with words and know each other's vulnerable points (which buttons to push), we have in our lives found occasions to disagree, and dirtily. For those of you with siblings or simply close extended family, you presumably know whereof I am speaking.

The style my sister and I have when a disagreement arises is to simply go for the gut right away, and make changes and corrections as the situation calls for. My brother tends to play the indignant card in first response attack or defense mode, and if that doesn't work, he will follow up with the hurt feelings or confusion card, with a final and usually ineffective anger card held in emergency reserve. As for my sister-in-law, well if she even chooses to get involve (usually we don't choose to involve her…), she watches the activity patiently and occasionally uses the back door communications gambit in order to express her concerns or suggestions. You have to understand, she really is a sweet woman, and usually just tries to fill in whatever needs there may be, <u>even to her own detriment.</u>

There is something else I should mention at this point: All of us were raised to be the first to throw ourselves on the barbed wire so that no one else might have to. That's an easier thing to do when one is young and relatively unencumbered by life, but to the best of our abilities, we still try. That leads into the further principle of "an attack on the one is an attack on the hive", or in other words, no matter what we think of one another at any given time, we will all come to each other's aid at the first inkling of trouble, and no one better mess with my Sis (or Brother, or whatever). Such can really mess up a good fight, or at least delay its conclusion.

A good example of the preceding would be a situation where my sister was attacking me fiercely (out of her depression as a caregiver) (It most definitely was not, I can hear my sister retort), and my wife, who had finally had enough, came to my aid against her. Good wifely thing to do, right? Not! All that happened was that my wife and I got into a fight over my sister and her motivations for starting the attack. It was not that I didn't really appreciate my wife being on my side, mind you, it was simply that no matter how big a butthead my sister was being, because my wife attacked her, I felt the genetic (or familial) need to defend her against my wife's assault. Now there was a real lose-lose situation, and in the end, my wife, my sister and I had all lost, and for that matter won as a result.

Now wait a minute you say, that last sentence was rather ambiguous. And that would be a comment to which I would respond that you were right. Nonetheless, it still remains true. My sister and I had a fight that as per usual ended in a draw, with hurt feelings on both sides and hopefully a little bit more understanding too. My wife and I were on the same side, but because of her comments about my sister, we were divided for a while, until we were not due to the mutuality of our basic positions; once again with the same results as with my sister and myself. Three losses, three wins, and when all was said and done life went on and nothing really changed, which from my jaundiced viewpoint is pretty much how most fights out there go and conclude. The exception to that basic concept would be unless someone brought an actual physically impairing weapon, but that's never happened in our family and let's just not go there…

Instead, let's get back to the fight (difference of opinion) we are all having, the things which are weighing heavily on my sister, (which include but are not limited to, over the last week: there being a leak from the second floor bathtub to the first floor kitchen, our mother's always perfect teeth needing to be pulled due to old age, my sister needing some 7k worth of dental work herself, the house a/c going out conveniently coinciding with a heat wave, and her working nights along with taking care of our mother). No real added pressure there, right?

I'll keep you updated as to how this all plays out, but for now my reaction was to endeavor to accede to everything she requested in her misery, to explain just exactly how, if necessary, we would be able to take her place, and to decide that from this point on, and warning all sibs accordingly, that all communications from this point on which concerned either our mother or the care giving situation would be shared amongst the four of us, at least those to which I was privy. Such an action should not only prevent any miscommunication or anyone being out of the loop, but also further minimize the damage done through lashing out at any single member of our four sibs in a cruel fashion. It also could shut down the sharing of innermost thoughts and feeling privately, but I think that might just be a loss we could stand. Time will tell on that.

The important things to remember from this chapter are these: We all care about our mother and want the best for her remaining time. We all care about each other, and hurt when anyone in the pack hurts. And we all want to help, and sometimes can't. If the person care giving refuses to be cared for, to accept the occasional commiseration, the odd kind word, the helping hand when necessary, however, then things will tend to become more burdensome on all, and most especially on the caregiver. Cutting oneself off from the help that is available eventually will lead to you the caregiver being overwhelmed by everything, especially loneliness, and then the loved one being cared for is not the only one who will have a diminished life expectancy.

Now, as to the update (a few weeks later and ten years after the fact)... If you are not an over-priced professional dispensing advice from your desk on high, and if you are personally well versed in family dynamics obviously the "let's keep everything out in the open" trial didn't work. It just made my sister madder and feeling more picked upon and isolated. This of course caused the remaining members of the sibs to feel compelled to at least give in to her stated demands of the moment and all disrupt our plans in order to get together for a family conclave as to mom's post mortem needs*. And very little was actually resolved other than that our sister-in-law who had handled such things twice in the previous few years should be in charge of selling our mother's house after she died (and my sister was able to leave back to her family in New Mexico). That and I suppose the fact that my sister was at least at some level able to feel like we would drop everything if she really needed us; something which was little enough in itself that we could do for her.

An Updated Update (ten years ago):

Well it is now several months later, my mother is still being cared for by my sister, and in Kentucky. My brother visited over the summer, and I did not due to the continuing friction with my sister. It is my belief (and one can certainly disagree with this point, that if my mother were to even be aware of a visit from me or anyone else for that matter and just for a little while after the fact, then friction with my caregiving sibling would not get in the way of my paying a visit to my mother. However, she is not so aware, does not know now that my brother was even there, and my sister and I have not found sufficient common grounds to make a visit tolerable, let alone pleasant. Hopefully that will change, but as of this update, it has not. Me thinks we are both losers.

*- No, it is not morbid; it is actually just a matter of realism that goes along with the scenario of dealing with an aging sick loved one. The house either has to be rented, sold or one of us has to move into it. My mother's stated desires of being gloriously sent off in a flaming Viking ship notwithstanding, do we burry her or cremate her? Do we hold a traditional funeral for a person who doesn't want one, or perhaps a gathering for friends and family with petit fours and Dr. Pepper in the park? Stuff like that has to be addressed, either in person or otherwise, (as strongly suggested in the Life Planning chapter), and that is at least what our sister needed us to do for her as designated chief cook and caretaker to our mother. Mom has a will of course, but wills for the most part only deal with the what, not the how, and the how is what suddenly was weighing heavily on our sister's mind, and causing her to be both needy and to lash out at us in her sense of being overwhelmed by it all. Like I said, it was little for us to have to do to help her not feel that way…

An updating of the updated-update:

Two years after the last update, my sister has been replaced by my brother in the caregiving of our mother. See the chapter called, "**A Changing of the Guard**" for how that went.

 An updating of the updated updating-update: No Viking funeral. It would have been one hell of a send-off however....

Cleanliness is Next to…..

Hygiene

Recently, I heard from a fellow caregiver the story of a sixty-four year old woman she'd been taking care of who had never actually learned how to take a bath. While this woman had been disable to some degree her whole life, when she'd gotten to the state of needing a caregiver, she was still apparently able to take a shower or a bath a couple of times a week, and everything *seemed* to be normal. Now there had apparently been subtle little clues, like even after washing her hair it still seemed to be oily (explainable), and the fact that even with more or less regular bathing there still seemed to be some skin issues (eczema, seborrhea). In point of fact, the only clue that really seemed to be unexplainable was the simple fact that periodically, everyone else in the house seem to get athlete's foot. I mean even the woman's doctors didn't pick up on it, and just kept advising and prescribing various topical ointments to deal with the problem.

In any event, one night after a particularly long dearth of this woman's not taking a bath, my friend offered to help her take one. Lo and behold the woman just lay there in the nice soapy tub and sort of ran the bar of soap around on her tummy. It shocked my friend a little to witness this, and so she pursued the matter further. Yes in fact, that was how this client took a bath, and a shower for that matter. Get wet all over, sort of move the soap near her body, and that was a bath. Whoa. No cleaning under the arms or privates or whatever; and as for the athlete's foot issue, my friend said the layer of sixty some years of old skin was like a foot thick (more like an 1//8 of an inch, that was just an athlete's foot joke, sorry), and so it there was an infection there it was certainly understandable that any medication applied to clear up the issue would have had a hard time defining it. The upshot is that bathing lessons were begun, all skin, hair, and infection issue were resolved, and the woman for a while constantly expressed how good she felt.

Alright, sure it was a somewhat extreme example. But as a caregiver, you are going to run into the problem of your loved one not wanting to take care of the slightly sagging sack which is his or her skin. Now there are a number of reasons for this. It's just too much trouble or effort for your loved one. It hurts too much to sit in the tub. It hurts too much period. And the number one reason, especially for older loved ones with diminishing capacities is: He or she is quite simply *afraid of the water*. In the above example there was, for years, a lack of knowledge which got in the way, but as time progressed, the issue of an inability to even perform the movements required also came to the fore. It went from not knowing how to can't do, and so thereafter bath time was a communal activity (and if you've ever given a bath, you know there is a certain truth to that line). Okay, and life goes on…

So what to do? If you don't bathe regularly or properly your skin integrity (and that includes hair) will suffer and all sorts of nasty things can result. In the case of those paralyzed to one degree or another, it can, and quite often does, lead into skin ulcers, and you really don't want to go there if at all possible. Anyway, there are things that you as a caregiver can do to promote proper hygiene.

First, No is an answer you should try your best to respond to. Yes, your loved one might not want to take a bath right now, but after a few days that can add up to a lot of past nows and missed opportunities. Find out of there is a concrete reason for your loved one not wanting to take a bath. Maybe they need some sort of cushion on the bottom of the tub to sit there with less pain. Perhaps you tend to run the water too hot or cold, or the act of getting into the shower or tub is perceived as too risky (they might fall or slip). For the easy reasons, there are easy answers sometimes like no skid strips, bathmats in the tub, and added hand grips on the walls. But what about the more complicated issues like actually fearing the water? What do you do then?

Constant reassurance can go a long way, and bribery might help too, but in the end, you may just have to get into the shower or bath with your loved one. Now I know that might be a bit embarrassing for you particularly, but have you ever heard of a bathing suit? Of course in the end, the answer to fear of water as well as some other reasons may simply be never to go near the bath tub at all. A properly given bed bath or standing in the middle of the living room as god made your loved one bath is a reasonable alternative to an actual bath or shower, and thirty seconds or so of warming up the water or bath solution will make it a more pleasant experience for both of you.

Now unfortunately, the real toughie that might come up is ultimately, the firm and no wiggle room dreaded no; The "I brought you into this world and while I guess I can't take you out but you damned well aren't giving me a bath" response. My mother got to that place, and my sister the professional nurse and my brother the towering male both couldn't really fight it. The end answer, well maybe you will just have to call in the expensive professional who isn't intimidated by virtue of being a child to the parent. The one they eventually found seemed to take over the parent role to our mother and, while still resisting, she did mostly acquiesce to the situation and take the bath or shower. Most states offer some sort of assistance for situations like this, and presumably they do check the references of the people they send. Not perhaps an ideal answer, but maybe the twenty or so dollars a week it costs will help you as the caregiver preserve some sense of sanity in the cleanliness battle.

Look, if you're reading this book, you care about the person you're caring for and want to do a good job. Your loved one does need to be kept clean for his or her own good, and somehow you will have to make sure that gets accomplished. As our population ages and more children take on the role of caregiver to one or more parents, the knowledge base out there increases and improves. If the ideas I have suggested for you don't work or you don't like them, ask around. Somebody you know in all likelihood is or has been in the same boat you are. There is an answer and you will find it if you keep on looking. Our family did, and you will too. Just keep asking about it, talking about it, with everyone. When my wife's mother was with us, we found that one of her work associates (my wife's) was in the same position we were, and they traded ideas about caregiving for quite a while. My brother was picking up things from friends all the time that relate to caring for mom. You never know what your friends and sometimes just casual one time stranger comments have learned and have to share, unless you talk to them. And hey, your work buddy might just appreciate the support more even than you do. We're all in this together, right?

I Never Tooted For My Mother....

Well in point of fact, it is the other way around. It is a known truth among my siblings, that in (my case) the first fifty-three years of my life, my mother never farted (broke wind, passed gas, and so forth). My mother was a lady, and after all, ladies just do not have bodily functions, right? Well since my mother's health has begun to fail, I have had a rude awakening on such matters. Has that happened to you yet?

To those of us who were raised by a modest mom or proper father, the very concept that they too have bodily functions can sometimes come as a real shock to our sensibilities. The notion that my mother occasionally has gas issues and can walk down the hallway like a trotting horse with the bloat sometimes is just not something which I personally, and I suppose my siblings had ever really consciously considered possible, and that leads me to the point of this particular chapter. Simply put, we are all physiologically build pretty much the same, and that which you can do which is perhaps usually not discussed, private, or even in some families *shameful* to even discuss, is probably going to arise in the love one you are caring for. As examples, I cite the following two situations from my own experiences.

When my father was in his last few days, the hospital in which he was staying was typically a bit low on staff. We family members who were there one night felt dad needed to be cleaned up a little, as frankly, he was slightly odoriferous. Now, it is important here for me to say that I was twenty-two at the time, the only medical experience I had had was with issues surrounding cows, and all in all in the world that a young man newly out on his own was typically in. Okay, I was naive.... Anyway, my brother took the top and I started in around the stomach area and went down. Mid way between the stomach and the knees is the part of my father I never expected to see, and as I got closer, I got more and more uncomfortable about my task. And then I got to his John Henry, his mother's little helper, his…, manhood shall we say. In my twenty-two years of living, I had barely seen let alone touched another man's *thingy* (a wonderful word coined I believe by Messrs. Python), and as I began to wash it, well it developed a mind of its own, shall we say. Boy was I grossed out! My father was unconscious, yet his, okay I will use the proper anatomical word now, his ding-dong got a stiffy! Whoa, was I ever not prepared for that one. Frankly I can't quite remember what happened after that, but I either immediately traded places with my brother or I quickly finished my tasks and then ran outside screaming into the night. Okay, while the latter was probably a quiet walk, I suspect you get my point. I found myself in a position at twenty-two that I never, ever expected to be in, and it freaked me out at the time.

Now, fast forwarding through marriage, my first wife's difficulties with her first pregnancy, the raising of two children, nursing school, and thirty some years, and we arrive at my next scenario. As part of my current wife's condition, she is unfortunately prone to something called "dumping syndrome". Because of the issues with her nervous system and simply put, on occasion, and thankfully there's only been two, her bowels can without warning decide to well, expel any and all contents. This happened one night in bed a few years or so ago, and as she in a totally mortified state woke me up at three or four in the morning, I stumbled into response mode. As she tearfully apologized for ever having done such a thing, her humiliation being plain upon her blurry face, I guided her to the bathroom where we cleaned her up, reassuring with the sure and certain experience of a man who had had two daughters and a variety of other animals throw up and defecate anything and everything possible on him over the years, that we had been warned such an experience was possible and that it was no big thing and there was no problem. When she was finally calm, I proceeded to change the sheets, sop up the mattress and disinfect it (no, we have a real one), and then deal with the trail from the bedroom to the bathroom. No harm, no foul, and we moved on.

Okay, so what do the two previous two situations have in common? Well frankly, other than being sort of gross and unexpected, not much. It's what they don't have in common that becomes important in this discussion. The major change from the first to the second scenario is experience and shall we say, familiarity, life experiences, if you will. Between twenty-two and my fifties, I experienced a whole lot of things which made my wife's situation much easier to deal with than the one with my father. The realities of my life now are much broader than they were thirty or so years ago, and so are my experiences. Generally speaking, that just comes with age.

In order to put that into context, let me throw this one out for discussion. Let's suppose you are forty and have been sexually active for years. The act of sex is hopefully a pleasant one for you, and you exchange bodily fluids with your significant other on a regular basis. You have therefore, experiences with the anatomically different areas of your significant other, and you are content with same. Now, suppose your significant other is now the person to whom you give your care, and it is the first day of your needing to wash his or her "bits". Changes things a might there, doesn't it... No longer are you involved with that part of your loved one which has been such a source of pleasure in the past, you are now involved with the cleansing of an excretory orifice on your loved one doing something to it which hitherto only your loved one had done in private. Puts a slightly different face on it now doesn't it. Then let's up the ante and make it not your significant other but your parent whom while you might have observed going to the bathroom when you were two, you haven't really since. All of a sudden you have a new and quite possibly unpleasant experience to deal with.

With parents and older relations, the mystique of their being human quiet often eludes a child, and the fact that for most of us they were somehow about as anatomically correct as the majority of production year models of Ken and Barbie is pretty much our norm. It is only when they become dependent on us that for most of us that fact changes. It is a normal response to be uncomfortable with such issues (there's a bad little pun there, sorry), but with *experience* and time, most of us will get over the problem.

A few months back, my cousin made the comment after reading some of this book that "Boy, you sure put it all out there…" Well I said yes, it was tough to write about a lot of it and thanked her for her acknowledging the fact, but in retrospect, I'm not sure if that is what she meant. She may have been chiding me for airing dirty laundry, which considering our respective WASP (white Anglo-Saxon protestant) backgrounds, is possible. Now I have not asked her, and I choose to believe that she meant it the way I took it (emails are so emotionless, so who really knows), but it would not be impossible for her to have been actually criticizing me for talking about things which people like us just don't talk about. We suffer or at least deal in silence about the darnedest things, and unless one is talking about children or is over the age of seventy talking to someone else over the age of seventy, the subject of bodily function is not considered proper for ahh, proper society.

Look, poop happens, as does pee, gas, drool, projectile vomiting (aka The Exorcist), and unwanted sexual arousal. Generally speaking, we don't tend to talk about it in our own case as well as in that of others, and generally speaking, we all engage in all of those activities at one time or another. The hard part comes in when all of a sudden, one is called upon to deal with such issues (there's that joke again) from another. No one says it is even pleasant, but it does happen, and for most of us, the more you deal, the less of a problem it becomes.

Another example: Somewhere in this book I mention our dying cat. Plucky little trooper that he was, he just kept going, and we loved him, but gee-wiz, he smelled like a porta-potty that hadn't been cleaned in months. Not his fault, it was actually his breath that smelled since he hadn't pooped in several weeks. But every time he got down off our laps after he required some petting, my wife and I had to wash our hands because the odor somehow stuck to them from his fur. Sure, we could have avoided the whole problem by putting him down, literally, but we loved him and he didn't want to go until he was ready. It's sort of the same thing with a loved one you're caring for. Yeah sure, you could put your saintly incontinent mom into the home or have a nurse come in every time good ol' dad soils himself and do the clean up, but if that's where you were at you would have done so. For some of you, I suppose it might still be an option for that matter, but not today, and not while you are trying to cope with yet another colostomy bag and its contents. Today you're simply looking for an okay that it is a dirty job but someone, you, has got to do it. So here, take solace:

"It's a dirty job, and you have chosen to do it. Kudos to you."

There, feel better?

Loneliness

Well, it's a quarter to eight at night, I just finished off a tall stack of Oreos and a short glass of milk, the TV is on the fritz for a few days until the repairman can come, and I spent most of the day cooking up some of the most tender barbeque ribs this side of heaven. The latter I did because my wife so enjoys them (I've never been that fond of ribs myself), the former I consumed alone because as quite often happens my wife wasn't feeling up to getting out of bed for dinner, again, and the middle part, well since I don't even have the mind numbing distraction of the usual shows we watch, I thought it was just as good a time as any to write a chapter on the subject of loneliness.

If you've been a care provider for a loved one for any length of time at all, you have probably already experienced the decrease in a life outside of your role and outside the house. However, if you are one of the many whose loved one is simply "not there" any more due to Alzheimer's or Dementia, or your charge requires a great deal of rest, quite often unexpectedly and inconveniently, btw, then you have probably also learned the Zen of just being there, ya know, in case….

Previously in this book, I wrote about personal space, and the fact that sometimes you would almost kill for it. Unfortunately, the opposite is also true. Sometimes, you can have so much personal space you feel you will die from it, or rather the loneliness it causes. If as I, you are fortunate to have someone you care for who is often around (but not always), you and he or she tend to develop routines together. Things like eating together at certain times, favorite shared shows on the boob-tube in the evening, you know, things like that. Those routines become important over time, even to the most unorganized of us, because it is during those times that you can share something together which bonds you together in some simple way. I mean you already have a greatly diminished social life, you may not be able to work any longer outside the home due to your loved one's needs and therefore don't even have a business persona to cling to, so in all honesty, it is those shared moments *together* with your loved one that can often be the highlight of your day. Unless, as with my night this evening, they don't happen.

In the science fiction novel, Dune, the hero says at one point in his travels that fear is the great mind destroyer (or words to that effect). I disagree with that assertion. Fear is bad certainly, but if you really want to get your mind destroyed, go with loneliness, it can be ten times worse. Now that's a fact folks, which is why so many prisoners sent to "the hole", would come out the most cooperative of fellows after a while. Loneliness was so awful, that the fear of ever having to experience it again was enough to make those naughty boys more placid. Okay, so you know I have to throw in an anecdote in most of these chapters…

I went from a family with four children to a very large college to a very large job to my first marriage where I helped create a family with two children. Now in the middle of those twists and turns, I was often a very solitary person along the way, shunning even the constant clutter of too many friends or activities which I felt often got in the way of things I wanted to do by myself. Ah-ha, you say, wanted it both ways, did ya? Well yes, frankly, and as most people do, I found myself somewhere in the middle of it. However, when my first wife and I separated, (our daughters staying with her for what seemed like good reasons at the time), I found myself in a nice little two room apartment with a lovely view of the St. James river, and alone. My God was that lonely… I went from being a husband and father of two straight down to just myself, and I thought I was going to die. I used to hang around the complex pool and office just to get a conversation in, and as for weekends, geez but they were long and tedious, and, ah, *lonely*. I suspect that's one reason I hooked up with my present wife so quickly after the divorce was finalized; I was just totally lonely and wanted someone with at least some compatible interests to share my time with again. Unfortunately....

  Unfortunately time passed, my wife has become more and more disabled, and I am getting more and more lonely (*he writes as his mind begins to once more wander to consider another stack of comforting Oreos...*).

So what to do? Well for one thing, I guess you could get a divorce or put "pops" in the home or write a book on caregiving... as for me, I don't see the first happening no matter what, because I love the old broad. You too probably wouldn't be in this position if you weren't in it for the long haul with old pops. I am writing a book on caregiving.

Now if the above three ideas don't apply, then how about bringing in a grown-up-sitter every second Tuesday so that you can go and attend that belly dancing class down at the Y (and if you've been eating those comfort Oreos, you probably have a big enough belly, you know). You might have those few family members or friends in for a game of Hungry-Hungry Hippos once in a while. You might even, (*dare I say it*), go past learning how to read all those Agatha Christie novels in *Slovak* and find new areas of interest in the literary world, if nothing else.

The one thing you can't do bucko, is stagnate like a seven day sucker until the next time your loved one needs you, or is there to share experiences with you. You may have to always be at hand, but for heaven sakes, find something to do that makes you happy for both your free time away from home and when you are needed at home, sort of. Contingency plans bro, they can save your soul sometimes. And if all else fails, ahhh, try World of Warcraft (*not a paid placement*). It kills major time and loneliness, along with Oreos.....

Now, **ten years later** (this will be a repeating theme in this book, since I was too lazy to just totally rewrite it in the past tense... Get used to it), we are living in a house up in the Sierra mountains, we still have the one housemate, have picked up another stray cat (housemate) who needed someplace to feel wanted, and so loneliness is now at worst a transitory experience. We all are in our own worlds for a large part of the day, excepting of course I, who is frequently in my wife's and our first housemates', a quick trip to town for a doctor's visit is about a two and one half hour mini event, and the local store for something forgot is only an hour less than that (I work very hard not to forget). Soooooooooooooooo, personal space is now more important than that of the issue of loneliness. However, as the two housemates are early risers and to bedders..., if my wife also chooses to call it an early night, I can get so totally bummed from being alone. Thank heavens for TCM and internet porn, right? (No, I don't the latter, but at least I know it is there...).

Of course there is one more point on which I have only scratched the surface previously in this book, and that is the fact that if you think you are lonely, imagine how your disabled or bed ridden loved one feels. You can walk into their personal space area. Can they into yours or for that matter anyone else's? Think about it for a moment. .... Okay that's long enough. You've got the idea, hopefully. As my wife just mentioned to me while I was doing this rewrite, sometimes she calls me in to do something quite simply because she is lonely. Get the picture? She knows there are times I am running ragged, and yet being left alone she get lonely and therefore might ask for my presence even though it is inconvenient at the time. Whoa; reality check there. I mean I already somehow know that, but hum. Maybe I need to spend a little more time with her when she wants it and not just when it is convenient to my schedule. Whoa, again.

Well all kidding aside, I really do try and give her all the attention she wants, but thank God for social media when I can't. She can kill hours of a day (I use that word regretfully, but almost all of us kill time at least once in a while), and she can connect with people who are actually happy to chat with her (and about the same thing she brought up with me forty-seven times 'cause she is unable to experience a whole lot that is new sometimes, and she is lonely) (Whoa, thrice). I am grateful for that facet of modern technology called social media, and you might encourage your lonely bedridden loved one to try it out. Just make sure he or she knows there are bad people out there who take advantage of lonely people and they shouldn't provide too much personal information. Do not assume that they intrinsically know that, remembering they are on a lot of drugs which sometimes clouds judgments. Then make sure there is top notch security software on their device of choice, and then pray...

Pain, Drugs, and Rock n' Roll

I arrived in the world of care taking and medications having once trained to be a certified substance abuse counselor in the state of New York, a position that I eventually left due to the following reason. It dawned on me one day as a smoker, that if I were unable to give up cigarettes, an addiction, who was I to presume to lecture or coerce others to give up their drug of choice. Now to be sure, mine was legal, theirs were usually not, and one can make a pretty convincing argument for pursuing such a calling despite being human enough to have an addiction of one's own. However, I didn't and still don't agree with that assessment, and while still believing drugs in general are something to be avoided, I do to my detriment continue to smoke. I take the requisite one aspirin per day for heart health and circulation, but other than that, except for the occasional need, I steadfastly avoid anything which will in any way alter my level of consciousness and for the most part abate all but the more potent of my occasional aches and pains. I don't drink, I've even cut my coffee consumption by half in favor of green tea for the anti-oxidants (a change which two studies thereafter suggested was misguided as according to their results coffee has more and no, it does not lead to colon cancer), and in general other than tobacco, I tend to lead a relatively clean and chaste existence. Which all rolled up together I suppose tends to brand me with that unfortunate term from my youth of being a "square".

My wife, on the other hand, a child of the sixties right down to being born and raised in the Haight (more or less), views illegal drug from a slightly jaundiced eyed rainbow-y perspective, and her own mega doses of pain meds as being something which seems to mitigate her pain more often than not, and so why not take almost all that is available. Well not quite. She actually tries very hard to limit the number of pills going into her body. Unfortunately, when pain is a constant, and the level of that pain is constantly high, anything she can do to get away from that pain is a desirable end in and of itself. I have come to the same conclusion, much to my internal surprise.

To be sure, there are those among our fellow men who take way too many drugs. They do it for the high, they do it for the low, they do it because they can't stop doing it, and they do it because as with my wife's situation, nothing else gives them anything resembling a life. There are a few barriers to such a life choice however, as well as reasons not to live on anything and everything one can swallow, and having discussed the need earlier in another chapter, this seems like a good place to talk about such issues.

Barriers to a drugged life fall into basically three categories. There are legal reasons such as the regulatory bodies won't allow a doctor to prescribe more than a certain amount of certain drugs. There are ethical reasons such as medical personnel who having never experienced chronic pain have no reason to suppose that what "x" is doing to a patient's liver is not far worse than what it does for that patient's freedom from pain. And there are sociological reasons that range all the way from societies viewpoint on why a person should be strong enough to do without and overcome to a caregiver simply refusing to give just one more pill at a given time. The last may be as often happens because there is due to the regulatory barrier only a given number of pills which will not be refilled before the next doctor visit, and for me myself personally, that's the one I have to enforce the most often. I know that sometimes my wife will benefit from another say, muscle relaxant, but I also know that even though she's put some back over the last week, she's also taken sufficient extra that she will run out two days before she can get a refill if I don't refuse. I hate myself for doing it, she hates me for doing it (and needing it), and this despite the fact <u>that we both know that I have to do it</u>; is a major bummer all around.

And then there's the question of the dubiously illegal, which is to say, marijuana. In an attempt to curb Mexican crime and induce more wood pulp usage in the early part of the last century, the federal government in its combined wisdom decided to make marijuana, basically a roadside weed at the time, the main focus of American anti-drug policy. Personally, I don't care for it, but for a commodity which so fuels the drug cartels and is so prevalent in its usage in this country; it seems to me the money spent to combat marijuana might be better utilized elsewhere. Don't get me started on the form of hemp used to make rope and whatnot...

In any event, marijuana is an (less and less) illegal drug that has soporific and pain reduction effects on the pains and conditions suffered by many of the legally disabled in this country, and has been proven to be such in more studies than can be listed here. It doesn't work for everyone, and admittedly there are many abusers of its calming effects, but still, why can't it be at least prescribed for those who benefit from it? Well the answer is simple, despite the various local and state efforts to make marijuana's use legal, it is simply that the federal regulations trump everyone's else's, and very few doctor's are willing to put their licenses on the line to do the prescribing. It keeps cancer patients from vomiting and allows them to eat, it has the effect of diminishing the intake of other more homeopathic damage inducing drugs, and it has the benefit for some at least of allowing an actual normal life to occur (to the point of no longer needing federal or state assisted living assistance).

The previous rant was sponsored by… Well as I stated up front in the first paragraph of this chapter, I was a trained drug counselor. I think people who take drugs recreationally are just plain stupid, but for those who have a need, my viewpoint has changed somewhat since my wife became disabled. With our prescribed drug bills we frankly can't afford her the luxury of anything like marijuana, and truthfully, my wife has gotten to the point that for the most part it just puts her to sleep. But for others, well I said what I had to say a paragraph ago.

On the subject of too much of a working thing; Drugs taken to excess, as just about anything else in this world, tend to have an effect on the human body. Too much morphine for instance, will make a person so constipated they feel like their insides are filled with concrete. That effect requires the taking of various anti-constipation drugs that may or may not work, and so on and so forth. Some drugs will eventually shut down your liver and kidneys, some will affect you heart or blood pressure, and still others will sap your will to do anything and everything. In other words, if a person takes enough long enough, the drugs ingested can ultimately cause problems that will kill that person. Ahhh, but there is a caveat…

If your loved one is dying of cancer, will in fact be dead in six months or two years no matter what treatments are taken, why the heck should they have to be in any more pain than necessary? I mean your loved one is going to be dead no matter what, right? So what difference does it make if his or her liver is going to shut down in ten years if he or she is going to be dead in two? Think about it. Most hospice care these days works on that theory. You as a caregiver are essentially that hospice care if your loved one has a terminal prognosis.

Oh, and since I mentioned it in the title, on to the subject of rock and roll. Music hath charms to sooth the savage beast (the actual word is "breast", but everybody gets it wrong). In other words, most people like music. Depending on their age group the type of music will vary, but to the disabled, it can at least temporarily remove their troubles and get them happy, to paraphrase the old song. In my wife's generation of late baby boomers, that tends to mean heavy metal and loud. But for just the merest of times, she is sometimes, when the mood is right, and the music is turned up to eleven, for a little while, almost pain free… Think about. Even a little while can be a blessing sometimes…

UPDATE: Now since this first writing, the legalization of medical and recreational marijuana has changed greatly in this country. From Colorado which lets it all happen from heavily taxed dispensaries, the rest of the country ranges down to a gram putting you in jail for quite some time, depending on the mood of the arresting officer and weather conditions. However, as previously mentioned, the federal government still has the final say, and as of this updated writing, it is conflicted, shall we say, on the subject. Just you and your loved one be careful for awhile longer, obey the laws of your state, keep an eye on the Feds, and just be patient. I would prognosticate that we all will be able to smoke very pricey weed pretty soon. Oh, and by the way, I never cared for it. Someone has to have all their mental faculties intact, right?

The, I'll Sleep Until I Die, Syndrome

Unless I don't...

Perhaps a bit melodramatic for a title, but you will see where I'm going in a moment. Besides, this is one of the shorter chapters, and one dealing with a subject which I felt should be touched upon.

People with disabilities tend to suffer from those disabilities, pretty much of a no-brainer, right? Unfortunately, they all occasionally suffer from things not directly related to their specific infirmities. Things like guilt for what they are putting others through, inadequacy for what they can no longer do, or at least do for themselves, despondency for where their life has gone; all sorts of normal emotions and emotions about things which we, as relatively healthy and functional individuals, can never really know. All the reassurance and support in the world may just not be enough sometimes and your loved one chooses what to their unconscious way of thinking is the only option available. They go to sleep. My wife actually has a name for it; the Garfield nap attack, based upon the kitty of the same name.

Now according to reports, my mother did a lot of sleeping. Twelve to sometimes twenty hours a day of sleeping, but she was in her mid-nineties with dementia, and just like little children, old people sometimes need the sleep just to maintain. It is obviously hard to schedule around, even meals, but one makes adjustments and frankly it gets to be just the way it is for some of our older loved ones. In any event, it is not those people in that sort of situation I am referring to in this chapter. I am writing here about people like my wife and our roommate who just decide one day that the only way to cope with life is to go to sleep.

Over the last few years, and currently as of this writing, my wife has taken to sleeping anywhere from sixteen to eighteen hours a day. It doesn't really matter what is going on in our lives or what special incentives I've managed to put in front of her (remember those trips I wrote about our taking up to Lake Tahoe), she just sleeps for most of her day, and for sometimes weeks on end. Sometimes it is to get away from the pain when no amount of medication will get rid of it. Sometimes, she suffers from ennui (on wee) so severe that her anti-depressants only seem to make it worse. And sometimes, well sometimes she is just tired from well, everything.

-Drives me crazy, especially when she repeatedly skips her doctor appointment(s) or some special meal or event I've come up with. However, with the passage of time as her caregiver, I have learned at least one thing. As with particular manifestations of her disease process, this too will eventually end. Yeah, it gets a bit harder to get what I believe is sufficient food into her. Yes she is missing quality time with me, her beloved (I get lonely, damn it!). But it *does* end.

Alright, you say, so what do I, as my loved one's caregiver, do about it? The best answer I can give is that as long as your loved one remains in good health, follow the words of the Beatles and *let it be*. The marathon sleeping will eventually end, you can finally read that new political thriller by that up and coming author D. G. Coe, (yeah, I've got one of those too), and things will eventually return to their relative normal.

<u>Now, as an important disclaimer here</u>, if this glut of narcoleptic (drug induced or not) activity goes on too long or if your loved one's health starts to deteriorate, *run,* do not walk, to his or her doctor or the ER and get some professional advice on the issue. Remember, I neither was a real doctor nor did I ever play one on TV. I am just one more caregiver trying to deal with life as it happens… Common sense does apply always, folks…

Why Should I Bother?

From Both Sides of the Question

Recently, I heard an interesting statistic which said that during World War 2, roughly 93% of a soldier's time was spent sitting around and basically doing nothing. Well, for the preponderance of those of you who have become fulltime caregivers, that is probably both the right percentage and the unfortunate result. Boring, you say; and yes it is. That's a lot of boring, er, boredom to deal with, and it has a really bad effect on your point of view sometimes.

Look, you've probably given up a lot to become your loved one's caregiver, and after the initial wonderful fulfilling moments you may have begun with (all that bonding and so forth), it's now five years later and you can no longer get by on just your self perceived sainthood and the gratitude of your loved one(s). Life has become a repetitious unending grind *of the same* interspersed by occasional emergencies and blogging on My Space looking for kind words from strangers (no I don't, I don't even have an account… yet). In my life as a housewife and mother (I'm old enough that fathers only did this stuff if they were single parents and until they got re-married), I cook, I clean (more clean-up than clean), I put out and monitor the usage of the various medications, I drive to the assorted doctors and hospitals, I try to motivate both physical movement and mental engagement, and… well the gratitude of my wife and our housemate (my other charge) is nice, but sometimes it rings a bit false and tiresome. In my free time, of which the is a lot between what needs to get done, well, I write stupid books (hopefully not), try and create art, and basically while waiting for the next need, watch a lot of TV and play video games. Damn! Once I was an international banker, a tech writer, and looked forward to the next day… Well I still do the latter, sometimes, but it can be hard every now and then.

So as the title asks, why should I bother? I mean taking out the whole religious charity thing and the family obligation thing and even the "there's no one else to do it" thing, really; why should I bother… Sometimes I truly don't know the answer to that one. The housemate for instance, claims after seventy or so years of living that he now so hates poultry (chicken and turkey) that the mere smell of it cooking makes him gag. Yet put enough fat, salt, and sugar on anything (America's top three food groups) and virtually anything with chili powder on it tastes good to him. Well he is an overweight diabetic with high blood pressure and so why try and cook anything healthy only to listen to the complaining about it while it is being eaten. There are only four of us in the house, yet now I have to cook both a turkey and a ham on Thanksgiving in order simply to have a pleasant holiday.

Neither my wife nor our roommate can be motivated into anything resembling exercise. Even the simple act of walking around our yard once or twice, something which they both used to do (albeit grudgingly) is now after years a thing of the past. My wife talks a good game sometimes of going up to the complex gym and using the treadmill, but it hasn't happened yet. Instead she spends most of her time sitting in her chair and zoning out on the idiot box between times of taking more medication (well, she does do more, but it *seems* that way sometimes). The roommate for the most part simply lies on his bed for the better part of twenty one or two hours a day, occasionally going out in his wheelchair in order to purchase food or cigarettes. Both only get up long enough to eat or use the bathroom. So why should I even try anymore? If I wasn't just too old and, frankly, too tired I should…

Well, taking out the easy justifications for not just chucking this whole caregiver role, I suppose the answer for me is this: First, I'm an optimist and frankly I like playing the long odds. With the advances in medical science like stem cells and pharmacology, I truly do believe there is a chance that my wife can get better. She's still young, relatively speaking, and if they could just figure out a way to repair what's been done… The pain would go away, the hopelessness of her condition would too in fact, and she actually might enjoy life again. _WE_ might conceivably have a life together again! And even if they can't fix it all, one way or another, just some improvement would go a long way to improving our lives, too. Hope springs eternal, and well truthfully, I do love the old girl…As to the housemate, well a job is a job I guess, and he does provide a companion for my wife, and gee, I do so love cooking chicken some days…. And then there is still the whole charity, familial, and last man standing aspect we were ignoring earlier. That's why…

So why does my wife bother to try and go on, or the housemate for that matter? I didn't know the answer for the latter, so I asked. Now keep in mind what has been mentioned earlier in this tomb, the housemate had an absolutely abysmal childhood, he's always been disabled to one degree or another with it progressively becoming worse over the years, and other than us, he has virtually no one who cares for her. What he said struck me a bit Pollyannaish, but hey, his viewpoint is so optimistic that it makes me feel like a dyed in the wool pessimist. Basically what he said is that despite all, there is just so much left in life to experience. He's seen things his parents could only dream of, like the first Black president and the Red Socks actually winning the World Series again. He knows that he might check out tomorrow (he was also fighting colon cancer, just for a change...), but he does too hope for a few medical miracles to enhance his remaining life, and then brother, watch out. He went on to say that there's just too much still left to be photographed (he's legally blind) and too many books left to be read or written. Me, I think he has a miserable existence despite our best efforts, but to him, life and all its possibilities seem to be still beckoning, even if I do slide some heavily salsa -ed chicken in on him once in a while because the money is running a tad short. Optimism and wonder seem to rule his roost, and that is why he still chooses to keep trying.

My wife's reasons are quite similar (and equally Pollyannaish). She chooses to keep going because there's more to learn, more to do, and more people she can help out there, especially those in her situation. She too of course hopes for "the cure" for her disability to one day pop up, but being perhaps a bit more of a realist than our roommate, she does know full well it may not be in her or their lifetime. But to her it doesn't matter. She has often said that she'd be happy to be the last one in line, just so long as there was an end to that line.

Alright, so in the end, of the three of us I may not be the biggest optimist in the bunch, but the things that keeps us all going, the whole answer to why we each severally and together thing there is reason to keep trying, gets down to one little word. Hope. It *does* springs eternal, it is why the guy or gal who came in second in the race runs another, it is why POW's and concentration camp inmates keep holding out, and it is why caregivers and their family charges keep on going, sometimes against all odds. Pollyannaish it may well be, but it drives the human spirit in all life, and *hope*fully it will never die out in you. At least I hope not.

Roommates and Housemates Are a Part of a Caregiver's Existence
unless you are independently wealthy
(*So you better get used to the idea*)

This seemed to me a good place to bring up a discussion of our housemates and former apartment mates, and their effects on our lives. Let me start with the easy one first.

Charlie, formerly Charlene (not his or her real names), is a transgendered female to male, sort of, permanently disabled old man who has been my wife's friend for more than forty years. He was tortured by her alcoholic mother, ignored by his father (who was gay, a fact which I think pertinent) and crossed the great sexual divide at least four times of which I am aware. Male or female, he has pretty much always been disabled, has Asperger's syndrome, has had cancer since the first edition of this book, is a diabetic by choice (as some diabetics are), is blind, has periodic psychological breaks with reality, has had two heart attacks and supposedly over two hundred strokes, AND, for the most part, he is one of the nicest people I know. He and my wife have been friends and apartment mates as mentioned for better than half their respective lives, he has been my client (State of California) for better than twenty years now, and has lived with us all of that time. There have been a few times when the income, generated by taking care of him and his SSDI contributions to the household budget, were not nearly enough to cause me to want to remain in that role due to his mental situation at the time, but once my wife went lame, that pretty much became a moot issue if we didn't want to live in a tent in a public park for the rest of our days. You need to remember, dear Reader, that my ability to work outside of the home and my wife's infirmities caused our financial outlook to suddenly become much bleaker, so Charlie's monies became essential to our continued semi-comfortable existence. Besides, due to his own actions, Charlie almost died twice, and I saved him with superhuman caregiving skills, so now I am his hero, sort of, and we get along much better now.

Charlie has seen more rock candy Christmases than anyone I've ever met, and as the song goes, if it weren't for bad luck, etc... His mother was also like his dad, gay, which certainly was not as accepted as it almost is today. She (his mother) tried apparently to forcibly abort him right out of her utero, (yeah I know, it's a uterus), hating apparently that she was not a man, and spent the first years of Charlie's life (Charlene at the time), making him suffer for having come out of her. His father maintained to the day he died that Charlie's mother *never* laid a *finger* on him, and so as you might deduce, the family dynamics really truly and completely were not hospitable to a normal childhood development. The abuse caused some of the physical disabilities, and most certainly caused a lot of the emotional and mental ones, and yet, Charlie is for the most part one of the nicest guys around. Give you the shirt off his back if you needed it, while at the same time almost killing himself secretly downing twenty or so bottles of aspirin for an unmentioned headache.

My job to prevent the last one you say? Well yes, mostly. But when he steadfastly demands his right to privacy in his own room, (to the point that if a six pound ball of lint is moved he will make everyone suffer for it), when he was able to go out and buy that aspirin himself at the store over time, and you didn't know it, whose fault was it but... I don't know, both of ours. The moment there was an obvious change of affect from all those aspirins, I was the one who saved him by getting him to the ER, but he never even mentioned that he had a headache, either to me, my wife, or his innumerable doctors. Therefore, while insuring his right to some sense of privacy, even his doctors having said that I practiced due diligence in my caregiving trade..., but still, we regularly tossed his room for the next two years in order to make sure it didn't happen again.

That was years ago now, and as mentioned in passing, Charlie is really a nice guy. But he has been on occasion a great deal of work which I could never fully get away from, especially so and completely so once my wife joined him in the ranks of the disabled. Oh, and the other time I saved his life was when the cat scratched him. That almost cost him his whole arm before it was over, and it was probably my wife's intercession with the doctors that has allowed him to continue being able to play a guitar. So other than financial reasons and the fact that he is a really nice guy, why have we continued to keep Charlie around? I will answer that in a few paragraphs.

Charlie 2, (Nooooo, that's not his real name either) our other and newer housemate, is not a really nice guy. He is just an okay guy if I must rank him at all. Charlie 2 was brought in when my wife went through menopause and she said that for the sake of our marriage, I had to leave. I didn't really understand what was going on at the time, and with two crips (disabled persons) in the house, even how it was going to be pulled off, but more on that later in this book. Suffice it to say that like the man who came to dinner and never left, Charlie 2 was brought in as the replacement caregiver while I was on sabbatical for six months, and he never left.

Now Charlie 2 is a nice enough guy I suppose, who seems to have no skills other than being a fifties era life of the party, (he never seemed to have left it), and who is about as useful as a bucket of air in a wind storm. Now that's not a very flattering description of him, but it is fairly accurate. He does have two essential features however, the first being a companion to Charlie, and the second, well he at least made sure that the other two ate something while I was away. He is old age disabled, which means that his disabilities are from the wear and tear of life, he is partially blind, has virtually no strength with which to do any chores, and we believe him to be at least a little autistic. He does not need a caregiver, but he most definitely needs a watchful eye if not downright supervision. He pays his own way most of the time, and is not a totally disagreeable person to have around.

So why do we continue to keep Charlie 2 around, you might ask, as you probably did a few paragraphs ago with Charlie? It's simple for the two of them, and very complicated at the same time. Because they have no place else to go. Let me repeat that: Neither Charlie or Charlie 2 have any place to go that would allow either of them to have a modicum of 'life'. Now you are probably sitting there holding your Rob Roy or Jell-O shot and saying to yourself, 'Huh?' Well let me explain, if that is at all possible.

I have now been a caregiver for over twenty years. I was/ am/ are still a parent of over thirty years. Being the latter fundamentally changed me as it does most people, and I almost became a good person upon becoming a dad. Becoming the former, however, on top of that, like it or not, changed me into something resembling at least an altruist. Hey, it may not exactly be my preference in size, style or color, but it is how life, God, or whatever one wants to attribute such things to, worked out. I could kid around and say it was totally a shock to me, but that's not really true. I have been, since reaching maturity at age ten or whatever, a pretty sharing guy, and so parenthood and then becoming a caregiver has pretty much shoved me the rest of the way into being an altruist. That's just the way it is I'm afraid. I mean getting older helps to be sure. I figure as you age you either become a bitter old coot or you develop a sort of, well, nonchalant view of things.

Charlie definitely has no place to go except a nursing care facility. He would probably, despite their best efforts however, probably die in short order too. Charlie 2 was living in a Veterans' home, and eventually would have died from his lack of wanting to keep living. Now they both have a place to call home which will not disappear or go away, and people who care if they are there tomorrow. My sibs think I am crazy, but what they don't realize is that they too in their own ways have also become altruists, (even if my older brother is a bit coot-ish, too). I guess in the end I am what I am, and I would hope that my kids will become altruists when and if I ever need them to be, too.

Oh, and as for my wife, well she has been an altruist ever since I've known her. Poor thing....

Note: As a general comment on the subject of roommates, apartment mates, and housemates, sometimes it Succoth the big green donkey ones. However, if he, she, or they are what God sent your way, (or life, or your coffee pot), then there must be a reason and he or it must feel you are up to the challenge. However, no mas Lord, okay? No mas....

The Art of Conversation

In the normal course of affairs, conversation is both a two way street and informative. However, in the case of that between a caregiver and a loved one, the rules tend to change depending on several factors. My wife for instance, has three main topics of conversation. They are her pain level, her physical condition, and the state of her bowels. Now all three are usually updated several times per day, if not in quarterly hour intervals, and if not for their constant repetition, might actually be informative. This is not to say that she doesn't talk about other things, but the more insular her world has become, the less she has to talk about that we both didn't pick up on the days TV viewing. And it is also not to say that to her, those three particular topics are not important. Her pain is a constant as noted earlier, her pain drugs tend to constipate her constantly, and her physical condition in general is the preponderant subject in her mind, accordingly. For me however, I figured I would be at least well into my seventies or eighties before the effect of a bowl of prunes would be something I would have to know about in a loved one. Well wasn't I wrong.

So okay, the above comments are not my wife's fault, but they do talk about a new reality I have had to face in taking care of her and which most caregivers have to eventually deal with. Whether due to diminished capacity such as dementia or Alzheimer's, or caused by an ever increasingly small world in which your loved one might live resulting from his or her disabilities, those long drawn out discussions on world politics, the prime rate, or the current hem length on which they used to wax poetically to your delight or disinterest, are if not yet, soon to be no more. Get used to it and learn to cope.

For those of my readers who have raised kids; do you remember how, when your children were little, your conversation devolved to something between their formative years and your intellectual ability? This is an effect well documented and even more pronounced in stay at home parents who at best might have actually interacted with other adults for a few minutes per day but for the most part lived in the world of "one foot, two foot, green foot, blue foot" and endless viewings of Sesame Street. It even became hard for them to hopefully go out for an "adult" night and not spend most of their time reveling in their parenthood and talking at a pre-school level to their significant other. And if you didn't happen to raise kids of your own, well you probably have experienced the condition vicariously from your friends or associates.

When dealing with a person with diminished capacity, the effect is more or less the same. Their lives tend to be in the past for the most part, and their anecdotes and memories often are all they tend to have. Whether from disease process or drug interference or simply a smaller plane of existence, your loved one may no longer has the resources to draw on for adult conversation, and so those things which are most prevalent in their lives, and their memories, are what they have to talk about. It lies upon the caregiver to accept this inevitability or if possible, provide stimulation to enlarge their world. And it further is the caregiver's responsibility to keep his or her own world from closing in as well.

One woman I've talked to, who is able to work, gave up her whole mother through great grandmother role almost entirely in order to become the caregiver to her own mother. She is able to work somewhat outside that role, but for the most part, she sits at home and interacts very little with anyone besides her mother and her mother's medical professionals. While not all that gregarious and outgoing a person to begin with, she has become almost as isolated as her mother in many ways, and after only a few years of being a caregiver, she is beginning to really hate her life. Not an uncommon situation to be sure, but one that she has made virtually no attempt at improving either.

In another case I know of, a couple took care of her mother who had had multiple strokes. The mother was basically unable to talk anymore, became more and more reclusive as the years passed, and eventually had to be placed in a nursing home due to medical necessity, just before her passing. This couple however, and who were perhaps lucky in some ways because of extended family, got the clue early. They didn't allow their whole world to revolve around the care of her mother. They maintained their outside friendships, they arranged for care coverage frequently enough to go out on dates and the occasional vacations, and they consciously created a lifestyle in which her mother was always encouraged to participate, rather than one in which her mother was the constant and sole center of attention.

So what did the couple in the second example do right and the woman in the first example do wrong? Perhaps it gets down to priorities in the end, because the woman in the first example had basically the same resources available to her as the couple. Even though she moved across the country in order to become her mother's caregiver, and even though she was no longer able to be an on the spot mother through great grandmother, she did have a life before care giving which she could have continued. She could have developed friendships with the people at her part time job which would have at least have led to the occasional movie night or dinner out. She chose not to. She could have continued her interest in "little theatre" or kayaking, or cat braiding, but she chose not to, once again. She even chose not to socialize with the family living in the area, except when they dared to visit, infrequently; the latter because this woman had become so wrapped up in her role as sole and exclusive caregiver, that she began to resent the intrusion of those family members in her little care giving world. Well more power to her, she will leave her current role eventually with less than she brought in, I'm afraid.

Honestly, I sort of understand the last part of the preceding paragraph. In the case of being the caregiver for my wife, I have created a more or less well structured little world in which we live, and one in which criticisms or interference have become resentments over time. And interference can mean such as recently occurred, the visiting of my cousin and her daughter (as per usual, as of this writing). For their part, they just wanted to swing by and say hello. For my part, my wife had had a particularly bad day the day before, was unable to find the energy to get out of bed and say hello when they came, and the apartment was much more cluttered than I would have liked. The resulting visit therefore was, shall we say, awkward. While I was glad to see them, as half of my marital couple I felt not whole, and edgy, and frankly, would have probably been happier if they had perhaps not come at all. I suppose I was also defensive, since as I was not exactly living up to my potential, I was waiting for one of them to say so. Thankfully, neither of them did. However, <u>all of my reactions</u> to that visit were constructions within my own mind, and I know it.

Getting back to the title of this section, in the above scenarios, I chose to allow my wife's condition to inhibit my socialization and conversational skills. The woman taking care of her mother chooses to virtually not have a life outside of taking care of her mother, and the couple, well in retrospect, they still feel like they could have done more for her mother now that she's gone, but at least they maintained something resembling a life while caring for her.

It is the caregiver's responsibility, not to give up living, and whenever possible, to stimulate the life of the person they are caring for. In the case of a loved one with diminished mental capacities, that second part can be particularly daunting, unfortunately, but it can be done nonetheless. If for instance, your ninety seven year old grandmother has chosen to live her life in the 1940's, then why not at least for part of the day go live there with her? Big band records, old movie posters and books about that damned man in the White House (one of the Roosevelt's) could be a great source of mutual satisfaction. Even if history isn't your thing, you might actually learn something (what does "all reet" mean anyway? What's a reet?). This may not help you become less insular in your existence, but at least it might broaden the subject matter you and your loved one have to talk about. As far as your existence however, well go back to the chapter on loneliness. It might help.

Music May Be the Food of Love,

But its Nutritional Properties are Questionable…

Chances are that the loved one you are caring for is on a special diet. Low salt, low fat, low this and low that, pureed steak and liquefied lobster. Old people and very sick people, especially with high blood pressure and lowered motility (the ahh, ability to not only absorb food content but to make and pass poop), tend to be put on such diets, and their reactions usually boil down to one of three responses.

First, they are wholly compliant with such dietary requirements, and present the caregiver with no problems whatsoever in their meal preparation or feedings. (So the .00943% of you caregivers out there who have such a situation, you may consider yourself lucky).

Second, they are wholly non-compliant with their dietary orders and go out of their way either out of eye sight or right in front of you sometimes to eat all the junk that they can. Such loved ones tend to spike blood pressures and glucose levels on a regular basis, and further usually end up shortening their lives and your term of caregiving, accordingly. Let's call that percentage about one third of the whole.

Third, there is the semi-compliant group, and make no mistake about it, part of that semi-compliance rests firmly on your overburdened shoulders. To a varying degree, this group tries to be good, tries to not crave that piece of chocolate cake which will affect not only their diabetes but further clog them up for a week *because that's what chocolate does…,* and only occasionally slips due to self will or determination. Your part as a caregiver comes in here in several ways. You feel sorry for mom because she can't share in her own birthday cake. You took a shortcut and used canned peas (lots of salt) for dinner instead of fresh or frozen. Maybe dad just so loved his bacon in the morning that you thought, well, just this once…… The fact that his arteries are so clogged up, well…. Let's also call this group about one third of the group in question.

Now wait a minute you say, that's only two thirds or so; where's the other third? In point of fact, there is one more group, a fourth third if you will, and it is divided into roughly two equal but different halves. That group is the "I'm not hungry" one and the itemized grazers. This batch is probably the hardest of the three groups to deal with, and if you can't master it, the members thereof will probably die from malnourishment. Now there's a cheery thought, but there's hope too, and we will address that fact in a few paragraphs, as soon as we deal with groups two and three (*we aren't even going to talk to group* **one** *anymore in this chapter. Big show-offs…*)

 Anyway, as of this writing (you've probably noticed I do that a lot in this book), we have a dying cat. Any day now, renal failure, IV's for fluid, and any day now has dragged on for about three weeks now. Now you have to understand, this cat has at best eaten a half of one can of cat food in that whole three week period, he is getting weaker and weaker as the days pass, but, and this is the important part, he AIN'T READY TO DIE YET! His eyes are bright, he still checks out his food dish which of late has anything and everything we can think of to entice him to eat, and he still, lord knows how, more or less (with help sometimes) finds the energy to jump up in our laps if only to sleep there in total exhaustion. The vet figured him a goner last week, we keep expecting him to not wake up, and well, like I said, he isn't apparently ready to pass on to that great litter box in the sky as yet. He doesn't appear to be suffering, and as long as he seems relatively content, we figure the decision to go or stay is pretty much his.

Now I mention the above for a variety of reasons, mostly though because our cat illustrates an important point: The desire to survive. Our mother seemed to have it, my wife and roommate both state it; but what exactly is it? Well simply put, it is a real or imagined belief that there is some reason to keep fighting, and frankly, until that is gone, there is always hope for survival. As relates to this chapter, that means eating properly, and despite statements to the contrary from your loved ones like "I might as well be dead if I can't eat...." or "I'll die if I don't get just a little...", it is a joint effort on both your parts to at least try and stick to the rules.

The first place to start is to not have around or buy that which temps. For groups two and three, if they are more or less housebound, that can solve a multitude of sins right there. So okay, you're still young and healthy enough to handle salt and cookies (which usually contain it, btw). So eat them someplace else, darn it! Gotta have that fat encrusted pizza with all the toppings and a pint of Cherry Hernandez (copyright issues) for desert? Have it for lunch or on that occasional night out (but chew some breath mints before you get home). The plain out and out fact of the matter is that your loved one's diet is your responsibility, and you don't want to be Eve's snake with the sugar coated overly salted apple; Right?

Now getting down to basics, let us state up front that salt substitutes don't really, and sugar substitutes taste funny sometimes. We all know that, deep in our hearts if nowhere else, yet along with a lot of fats, those (salt and sugar) comprise the true essence of the average diet. Please note here, I did not say the diet, but as for what compels us to want candy or Mickey D's or most of the stuff we have incorporated into our diets, the essence of our longings gets down usually to those three ingredients. So how do you cope? You can't stop wanting them in your food, so it is a little unrealistic to expect your loved one to either, right? Maybe it all gets down to compromise and doing the best you can most of the time.

Our third group of "trying to-s" is well trying, with your help. Sure you can do better, but if you can make a few compromises at least, and do manage to do your best, well sometimes that's about all you can do. I mean you're just human, right? And unless you've got one of those golden round things floating above your head, (like mine), you can only do your best, and that goes for your loved one as well. Doctors aren't stupid. They know that whatever they prescribe as to your loved one's diet, with very few exceptions it is just a strive for kind of guideline. I mean so all salt is supposed to be cut from your loved one's diet, and you decrease it by seventy-five or eighty percent. Hey pat both of you on the back for at least doing that much. Your insulin dependent diabetic occasionally sneaks a candy bar? Well in truth, I've never met a diabetic who didn't, even if only once in a blue moon. It all gets down to proportion.

Look, if you can only cut your loved one's salt consumption by ten percent, yeah, you're not really trying hard enough. But perfect is darned hard to achieve, and so just do your best. If you need the doctor to read the riot act to your loved one, do it. If you cannot live without a juicy hamburger at least once a day, then eat it away from the house (remember the breath mints), and if your loved one is semi-mobile and steadfastly refuses to stop eating a whole bag of candy or whatever at a sitting, well as long as you keep trying….. But then go and ask for help.

Now as to our fourth third group, this one is a toughie. Sometimes it pretty much gets down to trying everything, and bribes in the end; because frankly, if you can't solve the problem, eventually the doctor will start ordering IV's.

With my mother for instance, my sister noticed she was a light meal eater, but would graze all day and night if the right things were available. In my mom's case, that turned out to be oranges and other sorts of fruit. She (Mom) got her vitamins, so even though she ate her meals like the proverbial bird, she did do more. Two or three of those bags of oranges per week sometimes got consumed, because as her memory was so short, she would walk into the kitchen see an orange, remember how much she liked oranges, and eat one. That scenario apparently played out for her as often as every half hour sometimes. Hey, it worked, and it was healthy.

Not with others, it gets down to smell or taste, or both. My wife can have no appetite at all, but if I cook the right thing, and it smells really good…..... and then if I can get her to try just a smidge… This is not to say that my wife refuses food, she has a junk food habit on her shoulder for that matter, but… She also has low blood sugar and pressure, is losing weight despite a lot of her favorite foods, and I can at least get some healthy food into her usually before she hits the beef jerky and chocolate. Remember compromise?

In the end, sometimes you just can't win the nutrition battle. But if you do your best, then again, you might. Do what you can, hide what you can't live without; buy some breath mints if necessary. Just do your best.

Update: Well since moving to the country, my wife's physical status had worsened and her pain level increased accordingly. The net result was that she became mostly bedridden, and that meant she became a situational diabetic. Now what that means, it is simply that until she starts moving around on her own again, she will be an insulin dependent diabetic. The good news is that if she makes it trough two shoulder surgeries which will allow her to undergo two full knee replacements, AND then she learns how to walk again, and does..., Well then she will in all probability no longer be a diabetic. Of course then she will need some tweaks to her back surgeries, but modern medicine has progressed, so..... Keep your fingers crossed.

Wither Thou Goest, So (I'm terrified) Goest I…

I was talking with a friend the other day, whose two living parents are both in their upper eighties. He's one of eight children, and through joint familial effort, they have helped to get their folks out of their house and into a nice apartment more suited to their needs. His father is about as healthy as one would expect for a man of his years, and as for his mother, well she began to lose some of her marbles about ten years or so ago (that's *his* term for it). His father does a reasonable job of caring for his mother, and there are three in the area siblings who can take action with anything from a ten minute to an hour or so long response time should the need arise. All in all, the situation is more or less a manageable one as far as the parents are concerned. Unfortunately, there is one little hitch. My friend is scared that he will go the way of his mother and become non compos mentis like her (loose his marbled, too). All I can say is that there seems to be a lot of that going around these days….

My parent's parents all passed on in their sixties. My paternal grandfather did so around sixty-seven from a heart attack, as did my dad at sixty-six. All the males in my family have grown up with therefore a certain threat of reaching our end in our sixties. My older brother died way before that, but as for my eldest brother, well there was that quintuple bypass a few years ago… I guess he just missed his familial deadline through the advances of modern medicine since my dad's passing. He doesn't think so however. Rather, because of both that and his adult onset diabetes, he has pretty much decided (as far as I can tell) that he is near enough to his demise date that he has to spend the rest of his life worrying about it and when it will happen.

My brother and my friend are as you can see, pretty much in the same boat emotionally. Different reasons, lost marbles versus heart disease and whatnot, but both of them are to one degree or another, afraid of their heredity and what it may mean to their respective longevity. I suppose if it wasn't for the bypass surgery and the diabetes, they would worry about the same thing, vis-à-vis the loss of their respective marbles, seeing as my mother resided in the same sort of "Happy Place" that my friend's mother lived. (Now passed).

Heredity is a most wonderful and dreadful thing, I guess, depending on what's going on in the family tree. As a general rule, if the last few generations have been six foot tall blond gods and goddesses, then one tends to follow in the same height and beauty enhanced vein. If your mother and great aunt Ethel both had breast cancer, then there is certainly enough of a chance that you might succumb to the same malady that at least getting preventative testing seems like a good precautionary measure for your own peace of mind. If they also happened to be six foot plus blond goddesses in their respective youths, and you were too, well statistically the odds are therefore even more stacked against you. Please note the word, *statistically*, however....

Statistical probability is a pair of words as powerful as heredity is. One out of every two coin flips statistically should render the opposite side of the coin. If everyone in your background for five generations had either red hair and/or a fiery temper, then statistically a) You have a good chance of being red headed and quick tempered, and b) you should be grateful you didn't live back in the roman times, as I gather such people were likely as not (statistically probable) to be burned at the stake as creatures of evil. If three out of five of your male relatives had colon cancer, then your statistical probability of getting colon cancer is most definitely higher than that of the general population and you better at least get tested on a regular basis. So sayeth statistical probability, and so can be the curse of heredity. But….

There is also the other side of both sides of…., well for instance: Periodically, some mathematician will spend a great deal of time and governmental grant flipping a coin in order to prove the mathematical (statistical) truth of a coin flip being a fifty-fifty chance of which side it will end up displaying. Invariably however, they finish their trials with the result that one side or the other of the coin gets a great deal more shows. The funny thing is, that mathematical anomaly doesn't seem to bother the mathematician. Statistically the odds are what they are; the fact that one side displays more than the other is simply how things worked out. The statistical probability is still valid. Then there is the fact that everyone ever known in your family is a fiery red head, and you are blond. Well unless your mother messed around a little, and we will assume she was a saint, you just blew the statistical curve and your heredity, especially so if you are a very even tempered person. Chaos theory (I guess) two, heredity and statistical probability, zip. All heredity says is that there is a better chance that… All statistics say is that in all probability something will more likely be true is it was true in the past. And despite what insurance actuaries may tell you, it ain't graven on stone!

Look, my brother has diabetes. Statistics say therefore that my chances of getting diabetes are now higher. Okay, but his weren't, as familial memory does not give us any ancestors who had diabetes. My wife's mother had a bout of lung cancer, and twenty years later it came back and she died mostly from it. What statistics don't say however is that she also survived the holocaust and was nearly killed in it, and who knows what nasty chemicals she encountered while being slave labor in some of the factories she was forced to work in. There are no statistics for her family, they were all killed. So should my wife worry about dying from lung cancer now because her mother did? Should I worry about having a heart attack in the next fifteen years as my last hurrah? And should my friend really be worried about losing his marbles simply because his mother has?

There are no easy answers to the above three questions, but I do think there are mitigating circumstances to consider. First off, medical science advances. That which killed my father (etcetera) did not kill my brother because of medical advances. Secondly, there is nutrition and all that encompasses. My father as an example ate like most people of his generation. He got little exercise that wasn't forced by his doctor after his first heart attack (oh, didn't I mention that one, twelve or so years before the series of ones which did him in? Silly me…). Heck, the little red proprietary vitamins which most of us grew up on were barely on the table by the time I was ten. The truth of the matter is that he lived the life of his generation, and it along with the progressive deterioration of age and certain social, economic, and environmental factors did him in. My mother-in-law and her husband both went through the concentration camps and all that did to them and they died, he in his forties, she in her seventies. Somehow I doubt the veracity of my wife living in fear that she will succumb to the same maladies (besides, she said so), especially since her life is not theirs. Sure, one might make the case for her present problems being in some sort of a cause and effect relationship, but no, except for her smoking like a stove, she doesn't really worry about dying from the cancers which killed her parents.

Me, well I still smoke like my father and mother, he according to statistics increased his potential for an early death because of it, and she on the other hand died at ninety-three. So what effect do their respective histories at least as far as their smoking have to do with me and my smoking and therefore my chances of dying from something related to that smoking? It depends upon whom you ask and what they believe.

It is belief, or rather one's perspective on life that this chapter is really all about. Now somewhere in this book I've mentioned that all the health insurance money in this house goes to my wife. I therefore both have neither health insurance, nor can I afford to worry too much about that unfortunate fact. Yes, I may die tomorrow from any of a thousand different maladies, any number of which will be directly or indirectly linked to being a smoker and to some degree at least to my progenitors, but then again, I may not. If I spend all of my time worrying about that however, I will greatly increase the stress in my life and definitely pass out of this mortal coil sooner from the effects of that stress on my body.

My sister is now in a place where her post working age lifestyle is beginning to weigh on her greatly. While she remains relatively healthy at present (smoker), her position as our mother's caretaker and what that has done to her retirement situation made her already unhappy existence even worse. Every few months therefore she came up with a new plan for solving both her fiscal dilemma and being mom's caretaker, and every few months she came up with another one. The stress she had put herself under is something she shares in common with the majority of caregivers, and just like them, I suspect it will leave her in poor health in the end if she doesn't start finding a positive viewpoint from which to, ah, view things…

Now my eldest brother on the other hand started being sick in his fifties (the diabetes), had his quintuple bypass and was more or less forced into retirement before he was ready, the latter two being pretty much at the same time. He is ill, has seen the edge of his life, and he is also learning just how far his retirement money doesn't go, especially so with his medical expenses. A fervent ex-smoker (who does care about me), our phone conversations invariably contain at least one go-around on either my being a smoker or my not having health insurance. The result of which is that I verbally nod my head at his sage council and continue being a smoker and not having health insurance. The latter I can't fix, and as an ex-drug counselor, I guess regarding the former, I simply don't want to quit enough to do so.

The two of them together generate enough stress that I get a little stressed out worrying about them; much more than I allow myself concerning myself, frankly. I can't afford it, period. I would suggest to any caregiver reading this book that if his or her situation is similar, she or he can't either.

Look, the plain truth of life for a caregiver is this: You work with what you have. My friend and every single hereditary member of my family may lose our marbles someday. Statistically my brother and I, (and our nephews, grand nephews, and male cousins) will die before that affliction hits from heart ailments related to but not limited to smoking. But you work with what you've got. If my wife stabilizes, hell yes, I will go out and get a job with insurance (*and find out all sorts of things about my body that I probably don't want to hear and will worry about up and until the day I die*). But I will do it. As for now however, I try and remain positive about the future. What else can I do? If I keel over tomorrow, someone or some entity will take care of my wife. If I half keel over, then let's be honest here folks, how many people in any event can survive the co-pays which continue to go up seemingly daily with ObamaCare or private insurance. I/we will be financially behind the eight ball in either case. I therefore opt for a positive attitude for now and hope for the best, 'cause as I said, the plain truth of life for a caregiver is this: You work with what you got.

Caregiver's of blood family members are in the rather unique position of watching the slow and sometimes painful and disturbing deterioration which they too might face. Knowing that an errant gene may have it out for you as it does for the person for whom you are caring can be hard to take if you tend to be a worrier, and can also be just plain depressing, frankly. The trick is to bless it as it passes I guess, and if appropriate, do what you can to prevent yourself from succumbing to the same fate. Maybe you can't stop yourself from worrying about your family history of whatever, but quite often, at least you can gain some piece of mind for yourself by doing all you can to either forestall or minimize the threat to your own health. As I said earlier, while I may fall victim to my paternal line's inclination for heart disease, I do know that I am, despite being a smoker, infinitely healthier at my current age than my father ever was. Now if I could just quit smoking…

Post Script…

Now in the fairness of accuracy, after completing this chapter I sent it off to my brother for an initial read. He was kind enough to catch a few basic mistakes (mostly my deplorable spelling), and to a degree (as I expected), he had issues with some of my opinions about where he current is at in his thinking. As I said, to me he seems now to be overly concerned with his ultimate demise, to the detriment of both his ongoing life and future. That is a mindset which research has determined most heart disease and cancer patients seem to share in common, for at least some period of time after they have been hopefully successfully treated.

His response to me (slightly edited) was this:

I don't agree with your assertion. I might have died if I hadn't agreed to have the bypass - according to the doctor. My coronary arteries were in very bad shape. The operation is very serious and because I was split open at the sternum and then wired together, I will never be quite as strong as I had been. The diabetes is an ongoing situation which requires daily monitoring. The disease affects your organs, your blood vessels, your vision and other things. My heart problems were probably related to the diabetes. If I want to live a longer life, I must take care of myself. This includes monitoring my diet, exercising and getting proper sleep. I must also avoid stressful conditions. Probably a couple of times a week I experience low blood sugar and have vision and cognitive challenges. I also am easily bruised and take longer than normal to heal. But I am not worrying, nor am I terrified, about my impending death. Because of the operation, I then became quite aware that it will happen - someday. I also see it around me much more now that I am older. Five friends and acquaintances have died in the past 4 weeks. To save you and our sister from having to deal with my stuff, I am slowly trying to figure out what should be done with it. I am also trying to decide where or if I should be buried and what kind of a funeral should take place.

He then continues later on…

I will admit that until I exceeded 66 years, I wondered if heredity would have an effect on my longevity. Now that I have passed that age and now that I know I can affect my body's health through diet and exercise, I kind of expect to live several more years. The other truth is that the Norwegian side of our family has a tendency to live longer than the paternal side unless cast down by cancer. Dad's sister, however, is in her eighties. There is a reality, however, over which I have no control - aging. What will happen to me in that process, I do not know. Hopefully, I won't become a burden to you or our sister or someone else and will go quickly.

Finally he indicated that I was wrong about the lack of diabetes in our family tree, unknown to me my mother's brother suffered from that affliction. He also said I should worry about our family's medical history, because as a smoker and being overweight, I am therefore at a higher risk.

Okay, I'm getting a little stressed out, now…

Sex and the I Might as Well be Single Caregiver

Now just as a sort of disclaimer, we're going to assume here that if you are reading this chapter, you are either in a marital caregiving relationship or at least had a mutual status of "significant other" to the person for whom you are now caring… Or you're just curious. Anyway, there are two general facts on the subject of sex which are true of your new situation.

First, no matter how good or how frequent you and your partner used to "get it on", the situation has changed, and undoubtedly for the worse. Second, assuming your partner isn't suffering from dementia, you aren't the only one unhappy about it. While it might not be a subject either of you wish to talk about, don't kid yourself or feel singled out, both of you are now suffering from this particular loss, my friend.

In the beginning…... my wife and I had a rather satisfying sex life. Hell, for years it was almost a daily occurrence, rarely just missionary, and frankly speaking I was the one more likely to want a day off than she. (Ahh, no. I will not explain the first part of that sentence, thank you…). And then she began to go downhill.

We regained some of what we had enjoyed after her first surgery, but as her problems progressed, our sex life did not. Things went from almost once a day to possibly once a week to maybe once a month to where they've been for several years now, virtually non-existent. And don't kid yourself here, virtually non-existent is not at a level of even the worst of our couplings a few years ago. I'm talking a starving dog and a sliver of boner here, kind of situation. The best we can hope for most of the time is a little bit of cuddling as we retire, and even at that, turning to her side for more than a few brief minutes causes my wife a great deal of pain.

Now, I am not going to belabor the last point, but suffice it to say that as we are monogamous in nature, there really aren't a whole lot of options to explore. Simply put, she can't, and wasn't even interested for years until she was put on the right course of treatment for her depression. And me, well let's just say that I do only what is necessary to keep my prostate from enlarging…. (It's true, look it up sometime). I have actually and uncharacteristically developed the mindset that even masturbation is somehow cheating on my wife, this despite the fact that she has encouraged me to seek such relief. Plainly speaking therefore, this aspect of our current existence stinks! Period.

Of course there are others who have it better than us, and those who for various reasons have it worse, but as a rule, our situation is not all that unique. What to do about it is the question. Suffer in silence? Go to nudie bars or pros? Seduce your next door neighbor? Well, that depends on you and your mate I guess. The professionals and lifestyle counselors out there will tell you that in some situations there are workarounds for whatever physical limitations might be. New positions might be awkward at first, but practice does make perfect for some, and a drowning man can't be too choosey about the type of rope he's thrown. If you need say, a good spanking once in a while and your mate is in a wheelchair, well some people could be turned on by how that configuration might be worked out. Whatever, if the potential for anything is there, you two can either adapt or do without; and personally, I would choose the former.

If for whatever reason the issue is as dead a one as your sex life, well things can get a little dicey here. If you and yours have had an open mind set on the subject of sex, then perhaps there are avenues out there which you can explore. If you are both disinclined to discuss such subjects, well then I suppose it is up to you and your conscience to determine if those same options exist. My wife would I believe understand my exploring in those directions, but I just am not the type who could, ever.

In my freshman orientation at college, on the second day as I recall a sex therapist addressed our group. She asked at some point in her talk how many of us masturbated. A few of us raised our hands. She then said that as nearly as she could tell, about five percent of us were admitting to the act, which left about ninety-three percent of our group lying about it, statistically speaking. That included a wide range of people with an even wider range of social, ethnic, and religious beliefs, and even those of us who believed that we were going to go to hell or get hairy hands were still doing so.

I've never forgotten that discussion, and over the years, I've heard or read it repeated in various places and forums. The simple plain un-glossed truth is we all get aroused sometimes and we all need to seek relief. Your situation as a caregiver to your partner is what it is, and regarding sexual matters, you will have to seek your own solutions, jointly or severally. Just try and keep as open a mind as possible. You will need it.

Now as you know from my other chapters, I tend to try and end on an "up" or positive note. Occasionally, that isn't as easy to do as I would like. This chapter is such an example. But before you get all depressed and feeling sorry for yourself please remember this. For the purposes of this book this chapter has had to run the gamut of all situations from the best possible scenario to the worst. If you aren't in that latter percentage, (which statistically is surprisingly small), then there is hope for you and yours and your joint sex life. You may have to work hard at finding that hope, but it is there. And do keep in mind the situation of a pair of friends of my wife. Both quads, the solution involved a body sling an automated lift, and a little help from their caregiver. If variety is the spice of life….

Now, as we are sort of near the topic... kinda....

Menopause and the married middle-aged caregiver...

Yes, even disabled women get it, and if you are a female caregiver, well then this chapter isn't really for you. Well though, my wife TOLD me it might be... and chapter might not be the right designation, sub chapter, perhaps...

Guys, women go through a change around mid-life which last through various stages and anywhere from five to twenty years in the duration of those stages. If you have survived same, intact, well then kudos to you. If you are just getting into it, well you have my sympathies, no, they really don't enjoy it, and no they really can't stop what they are doing to you. The following four illustrations may help but are not remotely limited to what you **both** *might* experience; and yes, I am the artist and my wife even finds them funny... sometimes...

An Old Hand's Advice

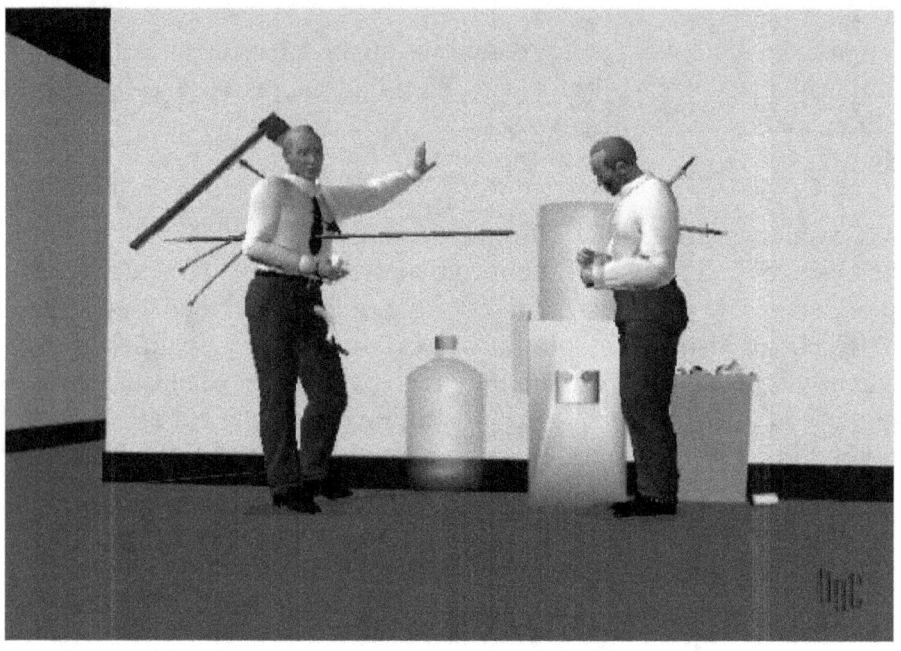

"So you say your wife has been menopausal for about a month now, right?"

Be Careful What You Wish For... # 17

For years, Buck tried to interest his wife in spicing up their sex life a bit.
She was never very interested *until menopause hit...*

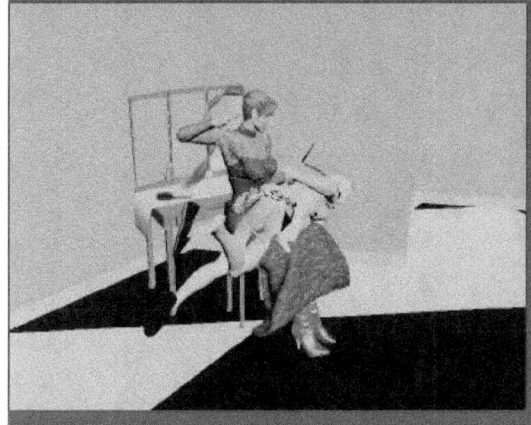

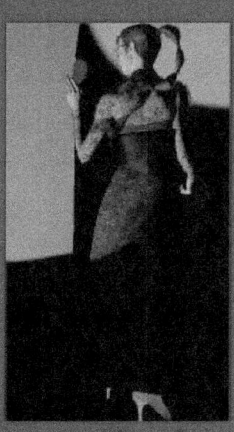

...and once you forgot to get the toilet seat down again, little girl, you will continue to wear this very little outfit for the rest of the day.

"Oh, and Sweetheart, if I catch you sulking, I might be forced to remember that this is bare-bottom day..."

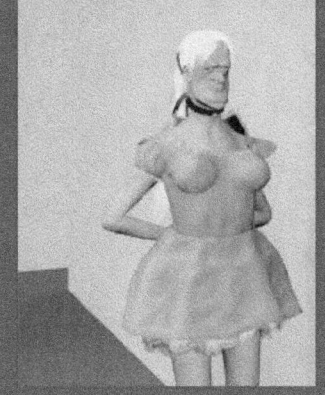

As he watched his wife leave the room, Buck knew three things for sure.

1) This was not exactly what he meant when he suggested spicing up their sex life. He just wanted to buy her some sexier lingerie.

2) All things considered, he sure as heck wasn't going to remind her of his idea for a threesome...

3) The dress and the fables were bad enough, but he knew she could have found a better wig.

DgC

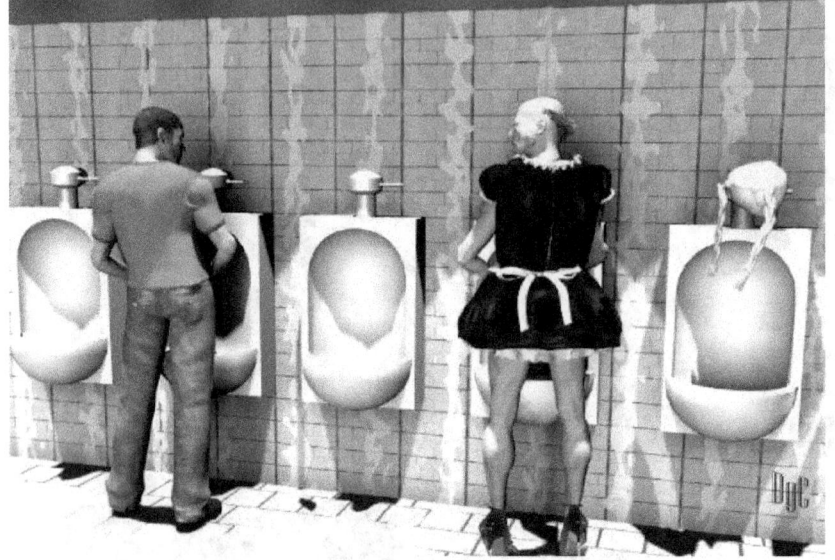

Because my wife's in menopause, ***that's why...***

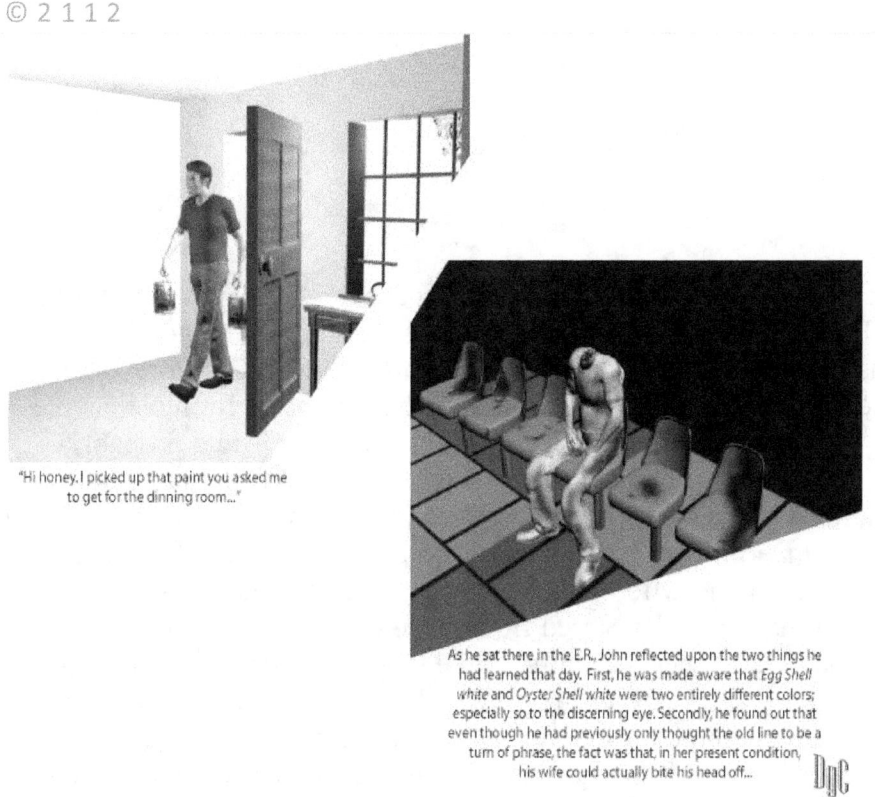

"Hi honey. I picked up that paint you asked me
to get for the dinning room..."

As he sat there in the E.R., John reflected upon the two things he
had learned that day. First, he was made aware that *Egg Shell
white* and *Oyster Shell white* were two entirely different colors;
especially so to the discerning eye. Secondly, he found out that
even though he had previously only thought the old line to be a
turn of phrase, the fact was that, in her present condition,
his wife could actually bite his head off...

Sure I do serious illustrations, but as for now, well, it's a coping
mechanism thing...... And if you think one or more of these hints at
emasculation..., Yeah, and???

Update: Yeah, menopause is now over. No, we still have no sex life
and I still don't stray. And do we both miss it? YES!!! However, it is
both of our beliefs that if the knees can be fixed (no knee caps), then the
pain will be greatly reduced and we once more will share our conjugal
bed.

AW, Come On Lord.................

In the grand scheme of things, after about seven years of caring for my wife I had become philosophical about it all. She had her good days, she had her bad days, and for the most part, she (and therefore I) both had relatively neutral, if somewhat less than the norm for most people, days. I had accepted that all things being equal, we would probably never see full daylight again at the end of her illness's tunnel, but then again, life in general was not exactly all black either. And then came the end of last December… My wife started to get migraines. Now don't misunderstand, my wife, like so many other unfortunates out there who share that malady had suffered from those particularly nasty headaches since I had known her, averaging three to four of them per year of our nearly twelve year relationship. She had had them since puberty, and usually they required a trip to the ER for some really strong drug to get rid of them. Such was her norm, and I had during our relationship come to terms with that regrettable aspect of her ongoing health. The usually preventative treatments not-withstanding, (they didn't work for her), the current disability and all of its drugs aside, we still made that average of three to four trips to the ER per year, and often around the time that most people are wont to settle in for a good night's sleep. This all changed on December 27th, of last year (2004).

As I indicated my wife got a migraine. It was treated, and that was that. Except, that wasn't exactly that. Two days later, we were back at the ER for another go around, and the day after that as well. In January we made nine trips. In February, twelve, and in March nine more. *For those of you keeping count that made thirty-three trips to the ER for migraine treatment…* Two o'clock in the morning, ten AM, they didn't hold to any pattern or apparent causative rhyme or reason. They just hit with little or no warning and required anywhere from a three to twelve hour stay at one of our fine local hospitals for treatment. And they do, (let's hear it), *as of this writing*, continue…

Anyway, as I write this in July, with no apparent end in sight to this newest of my wife's maladies, the count is somewhere around seventy-two trips and nine or ten successful home treatments. The ER co-pays are now up to about $3600.00, the doctor and medication co-pays perhaps seven hundred dollars, and we've just entered into the 2007 round of her Medicare Part D doughnut hole full pays (*you remember, the Republican Party's wondrous bootstrap help for the low income disabled and elderly which allows such societal dregs to fully pay $3600.00 of their prescription needs…*) (I'm so ashamed I used to be one…). Our net worth is getting redder, our more or less positive attitude of this too will pass is getting harder to say with a straight face, and personally, all I can think sometimes is, "Aw, come on Lord! Enough is enough! Geese….

It is at those moments of self pity (my wife just feels more and more guilty that she has been the cause of it all) that I try and put things in perspective and follow up with such thoughts as "well gee, at least we don't live in wherever", or "hey, we could have been one of those poor unfortunates on the evening news who just suffered through whatever"… Usually, that will cause me to join my wife in feeling guilty about what too many in this world would be an infinitely preferable existence to the one they are living. But sometimes, well sometimes it is just darned hard to know what to do next to keep our little family group afloat. I may even have to do the single parent thing and once more seek outside employment just to survive financially. This, while still fulfilling my role as paid caregiver to our roommate, and having to occasionally to some extent, hire someone else to come in at least sometimes to look after my wife's needs as well as that roommate's. And like those single parents, I will, as a result, just have to hope and pray that nothing at home will go *too* wrong... I think I mentioned somewhere in a previous chapter that the last time I tried that, several years ago, my wife managed to set herself on fire while trying to make a cup of tea, and she was healthier then than now.

It was a real conundrum trying to decide what is best for all concerned in such situations, and as you can see, as of that writing, I was still wrestling with it all. I have no great words of wisdom for you, my readers, and frankly, it's a toughie for me. I have opted to insert this article into the online version of the book because I believe there are those of you facing a similar predicament. I will update things as they transpire....

Update: And all of a sudden, the migraines stopped. The doctors had no explanation excepting something vague about 'women's issues and hormones'. It might have been peri or pre menopause, or not. It was just one of the wonderful experiences that make life interesting he said gritting his teeth and knowing that he was lucky it was not himself who had the migraines....

However....

Before I finish for now, I have a few mini-chapters to add to this one...

Ten Fun things to do While Waiting at the E.R.

1) Sit and contemplate your navel. On a longer stay, perhaps you might then try contemplating the navels of others.

2) For those of you smokers out there, keep count of how many people bum cigarettes off you in the course of a stay. Sub categorization can be determined by how many repeat customers you have, and during subsequent visits, how many repeat visitors you have (no, it's not the same thing).

3) Place bets on how many screaming babies it takes to clear out the waiting room. A variation of this theme is that of determining how sick your fellow ER-ians are, relative to their being willing to stick out that/those screaming baby (s).

4) If you, like my wife, are a repeat and frequent visitor to the ER, try and see just how many new problems (viruses, germs, parasites) she or you can contract while making these visits.

5) As you arrive at the ER, count the number of disabled placards in the disabled parking spaces. Keep a running tally throughout your visit for comparison.

6) Pick any given set of encyclopedias, start with the first volume, and see just how far you get towards the last volume before the reason for your frequent visits ends, one way or another.

7) A variation of number six is to just start reading the books in your house (heaven knows you can't afford new ones very often with your bills) and see how long it takes for you to run through them all. Then start on those beginning with the letter 'A' from the public library…

8) Play "car games" with your fellow detainees in the waiting room. I packed my grandmother's trunk is one of my particular favorites.

9) Listen to the conversations going on around you (not the personal ones) and when you see an opportune moment, jump in with a devil's advocate position to whatever the subject and point of view are. Do try to avoid getting into fistfights with this one however…

10) And number ten is…. Play ER personnel bingo. This leads us into the second mini chapter of:

The Four Types of Emergency Room Personnel

You might as well get used to the fact that all ER personnel are not created in the same mold. They have different viewpoints, different methodologies, and they may or may not let their personal opinions of you play a part in your care. The four types I will list are of course generalizations of many more, but suffice it to say that the treatment you get will generally breakdown into a fifty-fifty crapshoot amongst them.

Given a choice, which generally speaking you are not, the best two of the four types to deal with are either the "been there, done that" type or the well educated realists. The worst are those who are either judgmental or those who are in charge. In my wife's experience, at least the first two types seem to prevail, thank goodness.

Chief ER doctors are to be avoided. Regardless of their personal viewpoints on any matter, the truth is that they are the ones who have to deal with statistics and their relationship to licenses and accreditation issues. A good example of this is the doctor in charge of one of our former local ER's, who flatly has informed my wife that she cannot afford for her frequent need for high doses of pain meds (for the migraines) to draw down her department's statistics. The government looks too hard at her numbers, is what she is in effect saying, and it is better for my wife to go elsewhere's than for her pressing need to be treated in **her** ER. This particular one does have a way of preserving the billing process however. She administers the absolute minimum of drugs for my wife's migraine, and then having legally treated her, sends her packing. The result is twofold. First, we can be billed, and second, we simply end up in another ER and hope for actual proper treatment. This once stretched our usual four to eight hour visit to seventeen hours, by the time we finishes with the second ER. My wife's head by that point was pretty much lying on the floor…

The next type in line is the judgmental personnel, and this scans the whole range of those who might be involved in your loved one's treatment. The reason for their judgments are many and varied, but for the most part, the worst part of dealing with them is that on some level, you either know or have to wonder if they are in fact, right.

The other day, my wife waited roughly four hours in the waiting room, only to be taken back into the ER and be refused treatment by the doctor on duty. His reason: Migraine treatment was an inappropriate use of an ER. Unfortunately, he is absolutely correct on that point. However, as there are no twenty-four hour clinics in operation in our area, and as most of my wife's migraines occur after regular doctor office's hours, what choice do we have in the matter? The net result was, as above, two ER visits that night and two co-pays. However, this type of mindset doctor is fortunately a rarity in our experience, because while almost anyone who works or observes in an ER knows that they should not be used for non-emergency reasons (don't get me started on the billing costs to the insurance companies here), most of those people also know there is no other choice and go ahead with proper treatment. Such personnel almost fit into the "reasonable" category, but more on their traits in a few lines. Suffice it to say that, according to my wife's insurance company, egregious pain is an emergency and should therefore be treated in an ER when there is no other more appropriate substitute available.

The worst type of judgers in an ER, especially for people seeking pain relief, are the ex drug users or those whose lives have been negatively impacted by an addict. Such people will look at someone like my wife who already is medicated to the max for her normal issues, and say that there is no way she can need more drugs for her secondary issue of migraines. As I've mentioned before, I am an ex- drug counselor, and even I have difficulty with what my wife takes sometimes. The difference for me however is that I do observe her when she is not suffering too much and I see what she doesn't take and leaves back on those days. Yes, a lot of people are addicts and a lot of them go to the ER for their legal fix. But as my wife's doctor has flatly stated in several letters (which she carries) that she does need these drugs and has in fact both a high tolerance for them and pain, I bow to his more experienced and considered opinion. I just think so should the ER personnel as well.

Some do, which gets us to the third category, the "realists". Those are the personnel who have done their homework, know the difference between real and faked need, and consider the patient above everything else. Now don't get me wrong, sometimes they may choose to err on the side of caution and give a safer albeit lesser dose of drugs which may or may not totally fix the problem, but they at least do something to help. This group as far as I have observed represents **the vast majority of ER personnel**, doctors on down, and perhaps also the true spirit of the Hippocratic oath, to my way of thinking. Personally, I like this group the best, as does I believe, my wife.

Finally, we get to the "been there, done that" group, or perhaps better stated, the shared experience group. Such doctors and others have migraines, have back problems have whatever, and therefore have, at least to some degree, an idea of what the patient is suffering. If not, then they at least have had enough experience with others who did that their viewpoint is sympathetic. Such personnel are the easiest to engage with, they will sometimes get my wife in to the ER sooner, and they invariably will not let her out again until her migraine is, if not gone, at least nearly so. And frankly, it is nice occasionally, to have someone in her corner…

Look, I apologize to my readers for the fact that most of this chapter has been a self pitying haranguing against things we cannot control with her illnesses and against an unfair and poorly implemented healthcare system in general. But until everyone is provided with at least some medical coverage, until a safety net of sorts exists for everyone which prevents the loss of everything they have worked for due to catastrophic illness, well I just have to go on a harangue once in a while. I hope you don't mind…

And now for something a bit different (but this did seem the best place to put it...):

I recently met a man named Paul who had been, with his wife, caregiver to his failing mother. Many similar circumstances to share, but he told me one story which I felt was definitely worth passing on.

It seems that his mom had required numerous visits to the emergency room in a short period of time. He, like I, had made so many E.R. trips that he knew most of the staff by name, and he, like I was so ragged out that he could barely see straight. Anyway, on one occasion, he took his mom to the E.R. and she was admitted. He and his wife had worked their normal jobs that day, were short of sleep in general because of his mom, and he was accordingly just delighted to be in the E.R. at two a.m. again. Sometime after she had been admitted to the back, he decided to go see her and find out what was what.

Now for those .2% of you who are not familiar with the layout of an E.R., they tend these day to be set up in curtained off cubicles. Paul went to the first one. His mom was there, sort of... He went to the second one, and again she was there, sort of... Before he *actually* found her, Paul said he had seen *his* mom in nine or ten separate cubicles, and he was freaking out. He sought out one of the staff and told her that he wasn't sure, but that perhaps he needed to be admitted to the psycho ward because he might be going crazy. After he had explained his multiple visions problem, the nurse just told him to calm down because it happened to all of them once in a while, especially on busy nights. Paul was able then to calm down, but he told me it had a profound effect on him for a while...

I would suppose the moral of this anecdote would simply be, and....? But the moral is truly that with enough stressors and not enough rest, or anything else for that matter, we can all be stretched periodically past our sane points. It is how well or fast we are able to recover our sanity that truly matters, plus our ability to recognize when we *need* to ask for help, in the end.

Is There a God?

Alright, so if you've been paying attention, as this book has progressed, so too has it become less positive and encouraging. I could lie to you, my readers, and not put in the negative stuff, but let's face it; this book is in part a personal journal about what seems to be a never-ending and downward spiral. Now keep in mind here, my wife is not ninety years old with Alzheimer's, and I am still in what many these days would call the prime of my life. But the way things keep happening…

It had probably been about three months since I wrote that last chapter, and many things had happened. To begin with, my wife's migraines had been arrested, possibly through the judicious and dubiously legal use of what I have opted to call, "the California cure". Because of its semi-legal status, if you don't know of what I am speaking, then the best I can suggest is that you think of lighting one up in the Haight-Asbury district of San Francisco, and during the summer of love. Still no clue? Geese, you really do need to get out more, pilgrim.

Anyway, so her migraines were in abeyance, due to this alternative drug, and even her prescribed medications had been decreased drastically. Good news, right? Well sort of… This alternative soporific costs about half of what the legal drugs do, and its secondary or perhaps tertiary effect on my wife has been to totally remove what little drive she had left, for anything. That had caused even our few pleasures together to become virtually non-existent, and hasn't reduced our out of pocket expenses one whole heck of a lot. And I swear that the recent intestinal problems she had then were directly related to her new, "medication". The latter had meant that she also has virtually no interest in anything I can cook, but her desire for "junk food" has risen, accordingly.

Now, on top of that, I just lost a crown, she has a broken tooth, and the sum total of those two means that sooner or later, there is another two to three thousand dollars needed for the dentist. The regular bills just keep increasing, I may have to take work as a W*llm*rt greeter just to pay the bills, and I truly am beginning to wonder if either God exists or perhaps more honestly, if he gives a darn about poor little old us.

Yes, I know that God doesn't try us with anything more than we can handle, but when I look around at all the scams and double dealing going on in this world, at the profiteering going on by some off the hardships of others, at the suffering of the innocents in Darfur and elsewhere (Bayonne, New Jersey?), I truly do question my faith in a higher *benevolent* and involved power sometimes. I mean, my wife and I are good people. We give to charities, we try to help others when we can (or at least I do, she's too out of it these days…), so how come God has chosen to visit upon us the problems that he has? I don't get it. Unless something changes real soon, I will have to go back to work outside the home, putting my wife at a might higher risk, possibly making matters worse, and all because of things which in my youth I used to think modern medicine or perhaps simple fair play and relative luck would mitigate to some degree or another.

****

Boy, was I feeling sorry for myself the day I wrote that section... I left it in this book however because I felt it did realistically demonstrate that everyone has a bad day sometimes. Life isn't necessarily fair, but bemoaning the fact is something both necessary and transitory. God never closes a door but that he doesn't open a window, even it its only for a mouse's house... And that sentiment leads us to the acronym, **H.A.R.D**.

H is for the hunger you must not suffer,

A is for the anger you should avoid, (but can't always),

R is for the rest you need to avail yourself of,

and D concerns the depression that if you don't deal with the first three, you will eventually succumb to, and occasionally anyway.

Look to your higher power, your friends, professionals, whatever works, when you need help; take a walk, anything. For this too, whatever "this" might be, will pass...

Oh, and if you exchange the "R" for "L" (loneliness) and the "T" for tired, (**H.A.L.T.**). That's another acronym which leads straight to depression.

Remember at least one of those, and practice avoiding the effects accordingly. I suppose you could also go with T.H.A.R.D. or T.H.A.L.D, but neither of those spelling real words might make it harder to remember... Right?

 OH, and S.D.&R.&R., well you would have had to live through the sixties to know that one...

A Changing of the Guard

Life goes on, or ends, seasons change, and a few months ago, my sister felt the need to go back to her family and was replaced as caregiver to our mother by our brother. She was homesick, lonely for her children through great grandchildren, and absolutely scared to death (quite realistically in point of fact), that she was going to end up destitute if she didn't go back to work fulltime. She had been taking care of my mother for almost three years, and in the process had not only lost her then accumulated retirement, but was beginning to press at sixty with the full knowledge that she didn't have forever to work at her chosen occupation of nurse before her back and feet would both give out on her, permanently. She did her totally best at taking care of our mother and keeping her alive, happy, and safe, and I suspect will be convinced that on the day mom dies, it was somehow her fault for not staying with her until the end. Doing her best will not have been enough in her mind, and that self-delusional burden she shares with many, I am sorry to say (see end comment in this chapter).

In any event, in steps our brother, "Big Bro" as neither one of us has been inclined to call him, to take over the responsibilities of the caring for our mom. You remember my mentioning him in this book; the in his late sixties gent, the diabetic, the quintuple bypass guy, the one who as far as I could tell was ready to sit down and die guy? Well, funny thing there…., but I'll get back to that in a few lines. First let me draw you a picture of "big Bro". Sort of like the pioneers of old, he left the family influence early in life, right after college, and spent the next forty plus

years doing for others. From the Peace Corps to running several major
arts organizations, both local and state, he would visit the family
homestead (wherever it happened to be) a few times a year, just to stay
in touch and provide sage advice and counsel. I honestly can say that I
never really knew him until recently, my sister just a bit more, and he
was around so infrequently that since he for the most part prospered and
was happy, we all mostly enjoyed his visits and ignored his advice as
coming from someone who really didn't know enough particulars or us
to have valid input. I do think he and my father grew closer at the end,
and he certainly cares for us all, despite his perennial lack of
information as to who we are or at least were. Of late he is getting much
better on this last point, btw.

The important thing to remember about our brother is that for the
majority of his life, he has been a soloist. Other than a few cats and
dogs, and friends who have crashed in his home for various periods of
time, our brother has been a single man with no cares and no
responsibilities and no real interest for the most part in having either.
His work was his life, and his passions for living always were his first
priority, and he has never had the responsibility of caring for anyone
other than himself, ever. That is not to say that he hasn't been there for
others, nor spent his whole life being of service, but being unmarried
and childless does not lead one easily to being in the caregiving role, as
you might imagine. This life of Riley existence was further complicated
when I guess around 60, he first suddenly became an insulin dependent
diabetic and then went through his heart surgery a few years later. Oh,
and he was forced out of his job. The two diseases were undoubtedly
due to his lifestyle and heredity, the job loss was due to political
expediency, and his suddenly going from being a vibrant mover and
shaker to just an old ill man with mortality on his mind was not only a
shock to him but to us all. As I alluded to earlier in a previous chapter,
it is my personal belief and backed up by some of his subsequent

activities that our "Big Bro" was more or less resigned to his imminent departure from this mortal coil. And then the call came…

***

It was about a year and a half ago now that my brother and sister changed off in the caregiving of our mother, and I don't think my brother knew what he was getting into (hopefully he will someday pen a chapter or at least a few lines on the experience for this book on how it was for him). Now keeping in mind that our mother had become diminished into her own "Happy Place" at the time of this change over, and that her care on a day to day basis was basically making sure she was safe, rested and ate well; keeping that all in mind, you have to admire our brother for stepping up to the plate at that late juncture. Coming from virtually a place where he could, within the requirements of his previous professional life, suddenly pick up and go off to Brazil or New York on a moment's notice, and even retired do so as long as the pets were taken care of, to being basically the sole care provider for his physically and mentally diminished mother had to be a real head sapping decision for him, but he made it for the benefit of the "family", and we all have to give him credit accordingly. Heck, he even has begun to understand what my life has been of late, and that's kinda nice too…

I am now at the point in this chapter where I have to extrapolate about how things have gone for him since taking over from our sister, and guess somewhat at how he is feeling these days and how he has matured into his new role. I have come to accept that in our family, it is hard to talk about real issues, no matter how much we can wax prosaic and emotionally on side ones. However, in fairness to both my brother and sister, they can both contribute to this supposition as they will and have been invited. Due to my situation as caregiver to two, I have yet to be able to make a visit to observe anything personally.

My brother started out his new adventure by moving what seemed like about half his worldly goods with him, according at least to my sister and sister-in-law.. For him, that really gets down to his music, instruments, and accompanying paraphernalia, but it does apparently take up a lot of the little space in mom's house. Now one might perhaps think that was a bad thing for him to do, but in truth, what he did was move his own personal life and security blanket with him, and as a way of staying sane, it had its points. My sister left him detailed lists of every contingency concerning mom's care and well being, and between that, trial and error, and the further help of neighbors, friends, and our sister in law and her husband, "Big Bro" has over the course of the last year and a half managed to keep mom alive and kicking.

Now as far as our brother's life style, to be sure there were adjustments. First and foremost, he no longer had freedom to just pick up and do. When he wanted to go to an event last fall, my sister had to fly in and spell him for a few days. However, overall, he has managed to pull off the one part of caregiving that most caregivers seem to forget; he not only changed schools in mid year (colloquially speaking), but he further managed to join the basketball team. He therefore was the second member of the family who had to, *chose to*, totally uproot his existence in order to take care of our mother. He not only had to clean up and find a way to rent out his house, but to also put the preponderance of his things (furniture, forty plus years of stuff, etcetera) in storage, and at least semi–permanently put all of his home area local affiliations on hold for an indeterminate time, much as my sister had to do a few years earlier. Heck, he was even contemplating going back into the Peace Corp, a dream he'd held for a long time.

So he gave up a lot to make the change, but there is a bright side. He did succeed in creating a new life for himself after he moved in to become mom's caregiver. He has made many friends, joined a church, choir, and the local chapter of his lodge, and even found a way to finish off the course he was taking to become a deacon in his religious affiliation. That AND take care of our mother. Sure, perhaps her care did slip from a ninety-five under our sister to a ninety-two under him, but he managed to achieve the one thing she never could; being more or less content with his life. Considering where he personally was a mere few years earlier however, I have to view it all as a win-win for all concerned. Our sister is back in the life she loved. Our brother is flourishing in his new life. And mom is still *at home* and being taken care of by *one of us*. It makes me feel slightly less guilty for not being able to do it, despite my already full caregiving plate.* I cannot stress this one point enough however: My brother did build a new life in his new situation as caregiver, albeit a temporary one, and he is relatively happy. Anyone contemplating such a change had better heed his story, because as many others have found, to not do so can make the role of caregiver to your loved one doubly hard.

Yeah, so she's my mom, and this book is only a guideline for how it could and possibly should be done. I do feel a bit guilty that I can't do much to help in her care. Such is life…I take care of my wife and our roommate, my sister will I think feel guilty she didn't or couldn't stay with mom, and only people who have gone through this process will ever understand the illogic of it all.

The Fine Art of the Bait and Switch

As you progress in your role as a caregiver, certain issues tend to arise, over and over and over and over…, again. Hygiene, nutrition, simple movement in order if nothing else to keep working muscles ah, working; all of these things any many more concerning your loved one are now **your** responsibility. As discussed previously in this book however, all of these tasks are also not always easy to get done, especially when dealing with a loved one who has diminished mental capacities.

There are innumerable *legal* ways to deal with these motivational issues, some of which we have already touched upon, some not; but the one I wish to share with you here is a good method when all else fails. I call it the fine art of bait and switch. Now for those of you who have raised young children, you already know the basics: Sometimes in order to get those carrots down you have to put a little glaze on them or play "here comes the airplane". For the rest of you however, this may be uncharted territory, but it really is an easy technique to learn.

Let's suppose that Mary has a ninety year old grandmother who was raised on cleanliness being next to Godliness, but who has gone so far into her own world that even the how of taking a bath has now escaped her. While physically capable of taking a bath, the desire or even the will to do so has unfortunately gone. Mary, whose job it is now to get granny to bathe, and not stink (or have her skin integrity break down due to uric acid and fecal matter), has a problem. Ah, did I mention that granny also has a pretty good right hook? Well never mind, the point is how is Mary to accomplish her task, and do so in a relatively efficient and expeditious manner?

The easiest method in such a case is probably not going to work for Mary. Calmly and rationally explaining the necessity for a bath or how much granny used to enjoy a nice hot tub does not get through to granny anymore, because honestly, very little does.

Coercion is perhaps an option, but frankly, the paperwork is a bit much and who wants to go to jail for a bath, huh? Firmness is a bit better than that, but when you are dealing with someone who might actually be frightened of the bath water (like little children can sometimes be), it too is a method quite often doomed to failure. Me, well personally, I have found that the fine art of bait and switch or just plain out and out bribery will get results when nothing else will. So too did my wife.

When my mother in law was reaching mid-stage dementia she suddenly (to us) lost interest in bathing. We already knew she was having memory issues, and for a while we just assumed that she was spacing her cleanliness or perhaps doing it "European style" and just giving herself a partial sponge bath or something. We frankly didn't really begin to notice until mom-in-law developed an odor (our caregiving learning curve was slow and steep in those days). Well we tried various methods to motivate mom into bathing, mostly unsuccessfully, until one day my wife offered to help her. That worked a few times, but mom-in-law's mind was going, and soon enough we were back to square one. My wife eventually threatened that if she wasn't allowed to help mom bath, then she would call me in to be the assistant. Once again, that and the former worked for a while, but eventually… We were beginning to get very frustrated with the whole plan until my wife hit upon the fact that her mom had an incredible sweet tooth. Baths were then exchanged for desert or candy. Well that's great you say, but my dad, mom, daughter great uncle Ezekiel is a diabetic; can't do it, won't work for me. Ah-ha, I retort. How about fruit, or bergamot tea, or whatever floats your loved one's boat? How about watching re-runs of (eechh), Lawrence Welk? Something somehow will reach that core nerve of desire or interest; you may just have to work a little harder to find it. And if not…

We then get to the bait and switch technique. This was perhaps best illustrated to me the other day by a story my brother related concerning a recent hospital stay of our mother's. She is and has been as mentioned, now living in her own little "Happy Place", and recently had another bleeding incident and had to be rushed to the hospital. As per usual, the necessary procedures were performed, and the day following she was feeling fine, had no idea where she was, and wanted to go home. When my brother arrived for his daily visit, she was crying inconsolably, and he had no idea what to do. However, her nurse did. She asked mom nicely if she would help her fold some washcloths; that was it. Quiet, friendly, she asked mom to help her with a task that mom was familiar with, had probably done a few thousand times in her life, and knew even then how to do. The crying stopped, the desire to go home receded or evaporated, and mom was back to hr usual happy self. I mean the nurse probably had to go out and deliberately mess up a nice clean stack of wash cloths for mom…, but it worked.

Motivation is as hard or as easy as it is with a disabled or diminished loved one, and the trick for a caregiver is to keep trying sometimes until one finds something that works. No, any given technique will not work every time, but if you develop a broad enough repertoire, and chances are you will, then you're sure to be ready for most of the situations that come your way. One more example…

As stated, my brother is an insulin dependent diabetic. He was lucky enough to come across a credible sugar free fruit pie at the local supermarket. Besides being a motivation for him not to cheat his diet, it also turned into a staple for our mom. She has developed late in life a severe sweet tooth, and by happenstance, began sneaking into the kitchen and grabbing herself f a nice piece of that self same fruit pie. She apparently not only can consume almost a pie per day, but in passive coincidence is also eating better as a result. And it's sugar free… My brother didn't intend a bait and switch here in this case, but he got a good one anyway. Let's hear it for serendipity!

When Enough Just Isn't Good Enough

There are times in this world where, despite one's best intentions, regardless of how hard one tries, and irrespective of how much one has given up; one must sometimes end the day by accepting they somehow just were not what were needed to successfully see the job through. Such is not to be viewed necessarily as a matter of fault, as fault implies a matter of wrong-doing or insufficiency of action; for often neither of those terms is involved in the downfall of the situation. And even if fault per se can be laid, generally speaking it will be found to be on more than any one individual's doorstep, in the end.

For example, take the downing of that French plane off South America in the late summer of 2009. One can hardly blame even the most efficient and crack emergency rescue team for not saving the passengers and crew of that downed jet (although one young lady was picked up by a passing trawler, as I recall), because the last known position of the plane was not only far from the actual crash into the ocean, but the site itself was just too far away from any available rescue team. For reasons we probably will never know, everyone save one died in that crash, and it was to the best of our knowledge no one's fault. Bad stuff happens.

As of this writing, our family, and more specifically my brother is dealing with the fact that our mother has just been diagnosed with cancer. At nearly ninety-four years of age and with either deep Alzheimer's or some other mind limiting dementia, and being in failing health, the options are to deal with the cancer or not; the former being invasive, painful, and possibly life threatening, while the later could over the next few years end up in the same place. As our mother's current caregiver, the ultimate responsibility is <u>his</u> as to what happens next, since she is unable to understand for more than a few minutes what her medical problem is, let alone make the decision for herself. He has asked the family members for their opinions, but as the general on the front line, he and no one else will be the decision maker on this one. The cancer is very slow growing, but inaction for too long will end up possibly badly over time; however while surgery is definitely not advisable according to her oncologist, radiation and chemo-therapy have only a seventy-five percent chance of success (a one in four chance of recurrence), and both would make my mother's probably last days miserable.

What a heck of a spot for my brother to be in! Doing something doesn't seem to be the correct answer, and yet not doing something is equally fraught with potential failure, and quite often can be the harder of the two choices, as we all probably know. How this eventually plays out remains to be seen, but the one thing I believe can be surmised immediately is that no fault has occurred, that whichever action my brother takes could in the end be perceived as the wrong one, and that my brother will probably feel guilty for a fault which never occurred. As I said, what a heck of a spot to be in.

And then there is my own personal and rather unique situation. I have as this book details, been both a paid caregiver for our roommate, and also the primary caregiver to my disabled wife, the latter for nearly 10 years as of this writing. For the purpose of this discussion however, I am only concentrating on the matter of my wife. My dearest is now in her mid fifties, and in menopause, and it is that condition which has thrown all of our worlds into turmoil, plus one or two others.

Right now I am preparing to move out of our household for a period of six months, in order that my wife can determine if she wishes to remain married to me. Yet it was only five months or so ago that we were putting an offer on a house we had both dreamed of together (yes, it is still 2009); unfortunately, three things happened shortly thereafter.

First, the household cat scratched the roommate which ultimately nearly killed him and did cause him to spend nineteen days in the hospital pumped full of antibiotics. An unfortunate and unexpected situation for the housemate to be sure, but it also seemed to cause my wife to suddenly feel a sense of mortality for the first time in her life. Yeah sure, it happens to all of us eventually, but her father died when she was quite young, her mother died at the same time her cancer was found to be in a flair-up, and I guess she never got that sudden flash of "I am mortal" from anyone else in her life. But the housemate was different. He had been my wife's friend for nearly thirty-seven years; confidante, buddy, and on and off housemate; and the housemate's (Charlie) near death experience seemed to radically change everything for my wife. She started getting up early and staying up late, she went from a decaf tea drinker into a six or seven cup a day coffee drinker, and she began both writing again and using social networks for stress relief, a grand anonymous women's club, an audience for her efforts, and other things. She also started staying locked up in the bedroom for most of the day, supposedly to avoid conflict with both myself and the roommate, and that leads to or at least incorporates, numbers two and three.

For number two, it is sufficient to say that my wife's ego is so shot due to a variety of things including her disability, that the fact that our bid on the house wasn't accepted was enough to pretty much convince her that we would never have a successful bid accepted. On top of that add number three, menopause, and you have a great mix for emotional disaster. Some women go through menopause with a grin hiding a grimace, some with attempted manslaughter along the way, and unfortunately for a great many, for some with divorcing the most focal point in their external and immediate life, a nice guy like me.

Oh, oh, oh; I can hear you saying it as you read the last sentence. No, I don't kid myself, I am not perfect, I have made mistakes with my wife along the way, and since she has become disabled, I've even had to get downright parental to her once in a while (a lot). The last one I think may have been the biggest problem for my wife with her sagging ego, and I know it caused quite a few *loud* discussions between us. I will even admit that several times over the past ten years I have become so frustrated with the realities of our lives that I have firmly stated that a divorce was the only solution I could see. I also never went more than forty-eight hours before recanting and making up with the missus, either.

In any event, so here I am, about to be sent on an involuntary six month sabbatical from my marriage, losing both my home and my income in the bargain, and I don't really even understand why. A new caregiver (friend) will take over in my place, for the two of them (my wife and the roommate), I get to go to a family reunion which otherwise I would have had to decline due to their respective health issues, and maybe I even get some rest from my duties of the last years and my hair will start to grow back. My wife is going into therapy for women who are very menopausal and separated, and me, well I need to find a new place to live and a new job. I can guarantee you, my loyal readers that that job will most definitely not be in anything caregiver related; well at least I hope not.

Is this all part of God's divine plan? God, I hope so; but in any event, it is not exactly what I was expecting myself to be doing at this point in my life. Hopefully my wife will resolve her issues, hopefully we will find common ground again, I just don't really know. But it is an interesting turn in my personal life as a caregiver to be sure, and one which I will write about sometime in the future. Thank you dear reader for hanging in there with me, us…

Post Script (the inevitable one): Things have improved, I am back home, and I basically am doing most of the work the really old and tired replacement caregiver (Charlie 2) didn't seem to be able to do. To be sure, neither one of them died on his watch, but other than that, his main function seems to be reminding my wife how much she truly needed me by his ineptitude and inability to self start anything (remember I warned you before that you get what you pay for) The problem is that he really is a nice guy, but.... More later...................................... ?

 Later: It's been over a year and a half since we have reunited, and while life is improving, it also remains interesting. My wife has found some moral and more importantly renewed spiritual strength within herself, and I have become more pragmatic in my day to day dealings. In other words, the worst of the menopause is now over, and we are once more an almost unified (against the world) couple. Our housemate (Charlie) is now going through chemotherapy for the cancer she was diagnosed with early in the fall. He's resigned to it as well as she can be, even plucky sometimes, and the prognosis is good. As it is a new facet to the whole caregiving thing, let me just say that constant distraction of though and good eating are the keys to keeping his spirits up. Oh, and have a lot of comet on hand 'cause the explosive diarrhea that comes with chemotherapy is truly ah, remarkable.

Update: Okay, so the way the timeline in this book jumps around, if I haven't managed to confuse you, well then darn... At the point the previous was written, it was 2011, I think. I don't know, I'm old.... er... In any event, we were back together, in part due to the sudden passing of my mother, and we are now a family of four, as already detailed a few places in this book. Part of that is because my wife and I truly love each other, despite, part of it is due to altruism, and part of it is for financial reasons. In the next section I will touch on the results of my mom's death on my sibs and myself and wife mostly to wrap up the past, and then the new stuff for the revised edition. K?

Death and The Family Caregiver

It is unfortunately inevitable that there comes a day in the life of your loved one, when he or she passes. Now as I sat down to write this chapter, I did a little computation. My father died roughly thirty five years ago, almost two thirds of my life in the past. As I believe I mentioned earlier in this book, he had a heart attack, began to improve over two weeks, had a second massive heart attack, and then died a few days later. It was devastating to our family, but at least his suffering was short lived, and we all had the opportunity to see him in that transitional period between the two heart attacks when he appeared to be on the mend *and* lucid to make our respective goodbyes. He was the rock holding our family together, and it is probably fair to say that as a group we never ever really recovered; we just slowly moved on in our own and communal ways. My two wives never met him, nor my kids, and as for myself, well perhaps some of my mistakes might have been avoided had he been around.

My mother died a year ago last summer at the age of ninety-four. I was not there. For that matter, neither was my brother, her then current caregiver, as he had arranged for a little sabbatical with Habitat for Humanity while my sister took his place as mom's caregiver. The one thing I would like to get across about this whole time period was that if there is a God in heaven (which as you might have gathered I do personally not doubt), then he couldn't have orchestrated our mother's passing any more perfectly.

I had been away from my home for a period of time and had returned just two days prior to her passing. In other words, I was with my wife when we received the news. My brother who had done a good job of taking care of our mother, was in Africa with Habitat, and was surrounded by very caring friends and a few old acquaintances from his Peace Corp days. And as for my sister, who really carried a great deal of guilt for her not being able to continue as our mom's caregiver due to her own personal and financial issues, was there, at the end, and was able to cradle our mother in her arms as she slowly fell asleep and passed away. God's gifts to all three of us.

My sister, the nurse, was there at the end and able, I think, to have that closure with mom that she so needed. As a nurse she was also the best possible member of the family to have been there, as she knew the signs that indicated no, this was not a situation in which EMS was needed in order to make one more heroic rescue. It was mom's time, and my sister was able to be the most important person in the world to my mom, when she passed.

My brother, whom as I said was a good caregiver, would probably have, by his own statement, made that call for the ambulance, which may or may not have saved her for a little longer. However, in the end, I think, he would have felt extremely guilty that he couldn't have done more. He was as I've indicated with some very caring and supportive people when he received the news, and while still devastated, he did not have to deal with the immediate aftermath of her passing or the sudden loneliness and perhaps guilt that inevitably would have followed. As first born, his relationship was arguably the strongest, and his loss the most painful. God spared him the worst of it.

My reaction to mom's passing was loss, and frankly a certain feeling of relief. Her life over the previous few years had been constrained in that cloud of dementia most notable for the loss of a large part of her memory, coupled with periodic gastro intestinal bleeding and counter blood transfusions suffused with a total lack of comprehension as to why people were shoving things down her throat or in her arms and not understanding why she couldn't go home or where Dad was. Most of her friends and all of her siblings had passed, her life was quite literally in the ten or fifteen minutes surrounding the here and now, and at some level I suspect, she was at least occasionally aware of how much both first my sister and then my brother had given up in order to take care of her (not that either one of them ever would have said so). In her passing she was free of all of the pain and suffering, and in her passing she was with Dad once more.

I did not attend our mother's funeral, and many of you out there might think that such was just a horrendous thing not to have done. My sister certainly thinks so, and my brother is not happy about it. I can't speak for the rest of my relatives, as they have not commented. What I think I conveyed successfully some time ago to at least my brother however was the simple fact that I had discussed this absence with my mother some years before, and she had accepted my reasoning for not attending. My father's death was a true blow to me, and his funeral was one of the most unpleasant events I had ever attended. I say was, because when my second brother died a few years later, the open casket represented view of him was just so not the brother I had grown up with. Some people take solace from a funeral. I am not one of them. I prefer to remember my loved ones as they were and not as the dead body in the box or the ashes in the urn up there by the minister (etcetera) over which we must all get together to commiserate one last time. That's me, and my mother understood that. Had I been her caregiver, I would have gone through the motions for others as they required, but I would not have been happy about it. I knew that the moment she had passed she was with dad and her sisters and brother, with her son and her parents, and anyone else she wanted to be around. And yes, I will see her again, just as I will my currently alive brother and sister and wife and children once we've all passed from that mortal coil. I miss my mother and father very much, but they are better off now, so what's to grieve, right?

   This book, however, is about caregivers and their loved ones, so I will get back to that. I believe that both my brother and sister are glad they were able to take care of mom in her declining years. It cost them both a great deal, which they jointly pooh-pooh away, but they made the sacrifices with more or less open eyes and such are the results. At this point, neither of them is particularly willing to talk about the downside of it all, and any opinions I might have on the matter are just that. My sister-in-law does admit the loss, especially so as she had lost both her mother and sister (and her husband, my brother) in the recent past. And while certainly age accounts for some of it, I do believe that since Mom's passing, my sister in law has lost some of the spring in her walk, and is just a little bit sadder, as are we all...

We all are now the senior generation in our family, and we all have shared commonalities and differences which both join and separate us since mom's passing. Coupling that with the wild fluctuations in our economy and world events of the past few years, we all are more or less involved in our own personal quests for survival these days, and it is not always an easy road. My brother and sister are now through with their caregiving roles, mine is yet to be played out, and I hope to have my wife around for many more years. My brother is now trying to decide what to do with himself now that his interrupted retirement is back on track. My sister will work for a few more years I guess, and then someday she too will have to deal with retirement. I have more to accomplish for now, with my wife, my writings, and my children, among other things and considerations. I still haven't decided what to do when I grow up, but I have to admit I am beginning to feel a little bit older than I used to...

The remainder of this book will be devoted to my best attempts at determining what programs and assistance are available to the elderly and disabled on a state by state basis. In a few cases because of their size, I will even cover the programs provided in individual cities across the nation, as they can sometimes be a real step above those of the states in which they are located. Most programs these days are currently under the guns of faltering budgets, but it should give the prospective family caregivers and their loved ones a place to start.

In closing I would like to say that the writing of this book has been somewhat cathartic for me. I became a caregiver to my wife suddenly and without warning. The learning curve was steep in some places, and the costs were sometimes quite high. We almost went bankrupt from her medical bills, she happened to go through menopause just at the end of that issue, and for several years now we have been dealing with that problem. She is still menopausal (and that's been/is still interesting), she is still disabled (ah, duh...), and both she and I for one are still learning how to deal with it all. There has been a lot of happiness along the way, even some silliness (Passin' On Smiles, for one), and there has been some pain, well more than some but... Would I do it over again if I knew what was to come? Yeah, probably. And you know why? It is because throughout it all my wife has continued to be my one true love and best support individual. Despite her recent menopausal-ly induced lapses into insanity, she has always remained in love with me, and I know that even though I am her caregiver, she will always be there for me. It has been an, ahh, interesting experience, all around...

Is care-giving for everyone? Well I believe I made it clear in the beginning of this book that I really didn't think so. If there was a bad relationship before the need, then the care-giving situation rarely is going to provide for a happy ending. Even if the relationship between you and your loved one is a good one, the stressors and costs can and often are more than the relationship is able to handle. That's why I wrote this book. I am certainly far from perfect, but the things I've learned over time may prevent some of the negatives that invariably arise from the care-giving situation from becoming too harmful to you or your loved one. Jobs are given up which never can be regained, family members will invariably kibitz your decisions and actions (often negatively), and the worst thing of all is that an unending weight of complacency, loneliness, and even boredom can slowly sneak in from which you may never, ever recover. And if the latter happens, you, or at least your soul may die long before your loved one stops requiring your care-giving.

So tread carefully my friend. If you haven't yet become a caregiver, go back to the beginning of this book and take the test again. Maybe you will rethink your decision before it is too late. If you are now a caregiver, re-read the chapters of this book and use the reference section as often as you need to. Heck write a few chapters of your own if you want. Nobody gets it all right all the time, and no one will ever get it all wrong all the time, either. Oh and, good luck. I've had a bit...

And Now

For Some of the Stuff

Not Covered in the Original Version

Because it hadn't happened yet, for privacy reasons, or simply because I didn't think about it a few years ago...

Now, as touched upon in the rewritten introduction to this revised second edition, it is in 2015 and at the time of this writing, just under four years since the passing of my mother. It was traumatic for our family, it was after some passage of time also somewhat cathartic for our family too, and let's face it, we are all a few years older which by itself changes the way things play out in life. Charlie as mentioned went through a bout of cancer which I will shortly write about in length, my wife's situation has changed radically from where it was to a completely different set of priorities, and Charlie 2 has become a permanent part of our little grouping, despite his best efforts to not fit in. I will also write about that, along with a few other things which have occurred over the past few years and which I certainly never would have imagined would have brought us to where we are today, as of this writing in 2015. I believe that while what I will write might not be how things are now or will play out in your life, at the very least after your reading same, you might find some common ground upon which to contemplate our shared existence. It's good to know you're not alone! Accordingly, here goes...

Charlie and the Amazing Cancer Factory,

er, Repair shop

At the ripe old age of I believe sixty-six, Charlie the housemate was informed he might possibly have cancer. Now considering everything else that was wrong with him, we all kind of agreed that perhaps that was a bit unfair. Just a tad rude if you will, on fate's behalf, and absolutely not something which Charlie had ever wanted to hear. Well, it was what it was, decreed by God we supposed, and being more or less copacetic, Daniele and we decided to be good little cogs and see what the system had to give us. Two days later he had a colonoscopy, three days after that a removal of about nine inches of his colon, and two weeks later he started chemotherapy. Now my time frame might be slightly off there, but its close enough for this narrative, and besides, I haven't even mentioned the most important part of it so far. A diagnosis of cancer means one thing to someone who has never experienced it before. DEATH, painful, unyielding DEATH, and long and drawn out radiation or chemotherapy sessions which will probably result in DEATH! Oh, and since pinning an oncologist down is about as easy as pinning a medal on a gust of wind, while they all (the Oncologists, the Gastroenterologist, the Radiologist, and the Primary Care doctors) felt the prognosis was probably good, none of them would say absolutely. I mean they could have lied a little for Charlie's piece of mind, right? You know, said something like, "Well as long as it doesn't progress..."; but they wouldn't, to a man. Bummer.

So there was Charlie, a couple of pounds lighter, facing chemo after being told they had probably gotten it all anyway, and scared to DEATH about making it through the year long process and not dying. I mean he had quite a few surgeries in his life and lived, he went through the halcyon times of the drug fueled days of the sixties and lived, he even got scratched by the cat and not only lived but didn't even lose his arm due to septicemia, despite the best efforts of those little germs. But all of a sudden he was facing DEATH in the ah, face, with a disease which we all know of someone who died thereof and with treatment modalities which we also have heard are pretty darned subjective. Not a happy camper, there... Of course, in my Mary Poppinfresh sort of way, I pointed out that it could have been worse; he could have needed radiation therapy as well, but that little boon didn't seem to cheer him up much. He was looking at a year upcoming of twice a week visits to have some decidedly disagreeable cocktail of drugs mainlined into his body for two hours per visit, and a bi-weekly blood test in order to determine if those little cancer cells were succumbing to the poisons they were being fed. Hoboy, you betcha, good times there...

So what does a caring and concerned caregiver do for a person undergoing such an assault? Well first off, you better know up front that cancer or the majority of the myriad diseases out there that one can catch are not, repeat, not, generally contagious, especially so if they are hereditary. Ask your healthcare professional if you are not sure. Second, know and take appropriate precautions accordingly, that things like cancer drugs tend to affect your loved one's immune systems, and things which normally might have not been an issue, such as the flu, are now something to provide extra protections against. Adequate sleep, food and clothing apropos to the weather outside are vital to keep a handle upon, and so are things like flu shots and the like. If you are in a state where it is legal, pot can sooth a savaged stomach better than most things, and if not, well... Otherwise, have anti-nausea medications on hand would be a wonderful idea, and probably save your loved one some embarrassment and you some clean up, too.

However, the one most vital and important thing you and your loved one can do to assist in the achieving of a positive outcome is this: Establish and maintain a positive attitude; both of you. Do you remember that movie Robin Williams was in about a doctor called 'Patch Adams'? If not, go rent a copy and both of you watch it. It centers around the simple premise that the universal panacea for what ails one is simply laughter, and its effects can and have overcome the worst life throws at a person. No, laughter may not cure cancer, beriberi, or a car accident, but it can help a person through the treatments that can. My personal trick with Charlie when all else failed was to create three utterly off the wall personae with which to distract him. The drunken overboard and totally incompetent General Fubar was one of Charlie's favorite, along with the occasional appearance of both his aide de camp Major Malfunction, and others. One or another of them tended to show up on the trips to and from the chemo sessions, and any other time when Charlie seemed to need a bit of bolstering just to get through it all. I am as a rule perfectly willing to appear the utter fool to my wife and Charlie if it will make them forget what ails them. To do so costs me nothing, and done so properly and appropriately, tends to relieve even my stress to boot. In the case of my mother however, a different tack was needed. She didn't care for me to act like an idiot, so for her the tack was Scrabble and Cribbage, with the occasional game of Hollywood Gin thrown it for variety. In my family, games were the normal way of passing time and often interacting, and of yeah, normalcy is another key thing to try and maintain. Try and keep things as close to the way as they were before the medical issue or caregiving issue came into play. For my mother , she had spent fifty or so year playing games with my father. As the dementia set in, one way to forestall it was playing games. Something to think about, anyway...

As of this writing, Charlie is about three years out from that first scary diagnosis. He still has to go for six month check-ups with both the Gastroenterologist and Oncology doctors, but so far, so good. However, as each visit approaches (with their accompanying tests) we can see him visibly get more tense and more withdrawn. It is therefore probably important to remember that cancer even cured, is one of those diseases that will forever be in the back brain of your loved one, so you best be prepared.

Paper Cuts *or Being nibbled to death by ducks with egg teeth...*

There are some things said in life which one person says to another and which somehow are both hard to forget and quite painful. As a caregiver, you will be on the receiving end of more than your share, so you probably ought to learn how to sluff them off and perhaps consider the source. Here are a few of my favorites?

You're not living up to your potential

Gee, are you feeding ___ enough? She/ He looks kind of thin...

You know if I was the caregiver, I'd...

Maybe you should just walk away

What do you mean you haven't got the time to... ___ can't be that much work...

You need a vacation, to get out more, to... It not good for you.

If your ___ would just let you off the leash once in a while, we could...

You could get a real job. I'm sure ___ can manage for a few hours a day

You could get a real job. I'm sure ___ and ___ can both manage for a few hours a day

Oh my God, you look terrible...

And so forth.

The problem is, there is always a grain of truth or practical reality in most of such words of wisdom. Unfortunately, there is also usually a whole lot more truth and practical reality in taking care of the loved one you are taking care of, primarily <u>without help</u> the majority of the time. So, do the best you can to let such words not bore into you, and as I said, consider the source and know the offered advice was *probably* not meant to be hurtful.

On ObamaCare

The Affordable Care Act, or ObamaCare as it is more generally known, is a subject I have no admit I have no personal experience with. Frankly, that which was first conceived and that which was put into practice are so far from being the same good idea that it leaves me wondering about the motivation of the people we have sent to Washington to serve us and the country. Single payer insurance reimbursement, competitive bidding on a par with Medicare for drugs and services never even got out of committee for pity sake, and what we have been left with is a interest group gutted semi-national mandate which works, sort of... It may or may not be of use to both you and your loved one, but in my case, I can't afford any tier level that actually makes it worth having.

The affordable Care Act has thus far as of this writing survived two Supreme Court challenges. When the Administration changes in the beginning of 2017, I wouldn't make any bets on its survival. (Hint: There are many ways to kill a program if the people in power choose to... Underfunding is the one I expect will be used). Me, well on this issue I am a cynic, and expect the program to die. But hey, I've been wrong at least twice in my life. RomneyCare in Massachusetts was brought in by a Republican state leadership, and sort of works. And never forget all of those Republicans who have consistently claimed that they could put in a better universal health care plan than The Affordable Care Act. There just never seemed to be any details...

Look, the poor and working poor now have something, and it's better than nothing. The rich always will. In other words, the Haves and the Have-nots are pretty well set, at least for now.. Being firmly entrenched in the middle class, I look forward to Medicare and perhaps a supplemental insurance plan. And if as the only one in our household who doesn't have insurance, I become incapacitated, then well there's always Medical (California's version of Medicaid)... God seems to be helping me stay healthy until then...

If it weren't for God's faith in us...

... Then perhaps things would have worked out differently. Since the first version of this book, my wife is no longer menopausal, and she has started her second Saturn return (for you astrological buffs). Those two things put together mean that our life together has become much stronger, and we even somehow fulfilled the prediction of an Indian Shaman in Gallup New Mexico in 1995. If you are interested (and even if you are not), we met this intoxicated gentleman while passing through on our way to California, who said very definitely that we would separate for a period in the second decade of our being together and that we would get back together around six months later and have an even stronger relationship than we did before. I mean **wow**, that really did happen, right? I mean ancient Native American mysteries are mysterious..., so ya know....

Truthfully, I suppose that might be explained away through statistical probability analysis, but I thought I'd throw it in for human interest if nothing else. It is also a lite and totally unrelated way of introducing you to the next part of our lives together, which some might say is just icing on the caregiving cake, for a family caregiver and his loved one.

A few years ago, my wife's primary doctor was slightly concerned with the look of my wife's knees, and so he sent her for tests. It seems that she was losing her kneecaps and joints, probably due to a side effect of her disease process. Well, two things resulted from that. First he sent her to one of the best orthopedists in the bay area, who declared A)- (and this really is a quote) that yes my wife's knees were messed up badly, and that B)- he was not inclined to operate since she had a wheelchair and didn't do much walking anyway, so why bother? We were livid, but as he was 'one of the best', we just assumed that there was nothing really to be done. Besides, her primary retired about that time, and the practice became one more of efficiency than of knowing who a patient was. As most disabled people out there know (as do their caregivers), there are regretfully a fair percentage of practices out there who are like that, mostly due to how much care, paperwork, and time they must undergo and spend just to get paid by the insurance companies.

Now the second thing that happened was instigated by our moving into a lovely home in the Sierras, and therefore into a less hectic and overworked medical community. My wife's new primary noticed the same thing as her previous, sent her for the same tests and referral, and the new orthopedist took one look and said that they had in the ensuing two years that had passed, so deteriorated that if something was done soon, she would positively never walk again. Now we are not stupid, we double checked before going with his prognosis, and so the impetus went from worrying about my wife's back (with the five surgeries) to getting her knees fixed. Are you with me so far?

In the course of dealing with her knees which anyone could tell was necessary from reading her x-rays and MRI's, it was determined that she would have to undergo rotator cuff replacement on both shoulders, because they too had deteriorated and begun to hurt, and because she would never be able to uses crutches in order to recover from the knee surgery unless they were fixed first. You may also add to that the fact that due to her basically being bedridden because the pain of no knees (its straight bone on bone right now) she developed diabetes, and because she is violently allergic to Metformin, she is now on insulin once a day to keep her sugars in check.

Anyway, we are still in process towards getting the knees fixed, the first shortly after this revised tome is published, and Murphy's Law being what it is... Both shoulders have been repaired and the first knee was scheduled for being replaced about three months ago. Except it wasn't. The second should had to be fixed a second time because the day she had its surgery and came home from the hospital (out-patient), Charlie had a med reaction, started to pass out and fall, and guess who tried to catch him and prevent serious damage? Yup, you got it. My wife changed her 35% successful repair into a 95% third surgery some several months later which delayed the first knee. Well, my wife is plucky, I almost never say die, and that is how things are, as of this writing, for us. It is also however why I titled this chapter the way I did. I mean He, She, or It (depending on your belief system) must truly believe we are capable folks and able to weather almost everything, because when all this is over, she will still need some microsurgical repair work done on several of her previous back operations (the advances in modern medicine are amazing).

So, other than providing an update to where we were at the end of the first book, why am I writing all about this. It's simple. WE have as a couple become both pragmatic and hopeful for a better day. WE accept that bad things happen to good people, and that all of this is not for naught. And besides, we don't really believe in suicide. -Too much paperwork. Oh, and one more thing: Legal and semi-legal drugs are now a specialty in the medical community, and the previous prevailing viewpoints about same are rapidly falling by the wayside. It is a slow process, but most doctors and medical professionals are beginning to accept the point of view that pain *in and of itself* is a debilitating process, and the alleviating thereof is not a bad thing. It actually helps. As an extreme but pertinent example: If your loved one is going to die of cancer or Alzheimer's or whatever in six months, then what's the harm in letting them go comfortably. In my wife's case, she actually amazes the doctors with the level of drugs she allows herself to take as compared to what is prescribed for her. They know what the statistical level of medications is that she should be taking for her pain, and she consistently undertakes them to the extent that they frequently chide her for taking too little. Why, because those drugs also ameliorate her mental capacities, and she doesn't like it. Besides, they aren't particularly good for her kidneys, liver, or gastrointestinal tract either. I t would be nice if the underlying causes of her pains could be eliminated, but in truth they probably never really will, if for no better reason than that she is getting older and old people have aches and pains which will never go away.

Now it is true that some people will never be able to get enough pain killers or muscle relaxants to keep them happy, but that is a matter for them and their doctors to work out. If such a person is your loved one, then it is your job to determine if they truly need the relief or are simply abusing the meds, and to act accordingly as their caregiver. As a former substance abuse counselor, I can only offer that as a base point from which to assess your loved one, and say that professional help is out there, usually. Oh, and this too: Sometimes you can't fix that problem, only they can. You need to know the difference. I know it for my wife and trust her doctors to know it, too. And sometimes for your own sanity and health, you just have to walk away.

That leads me to something I decided not to reveal in the first version of this book. It is only time and reconciliation with myself that allows me to mention it now. My mother was an alcoholic.

Aha, you might be saying. So that's why... Well maybe. It did certainly affect my upbringing and the relationships with my siblings. Alcoholism is a disease process, as compared to heavy drinking which is drug abuse. It is that knowledge which causes me to be at rest with my mother and my life with her. It was not, I believe, her fault, it was a disease to which she succumbed. The results don't change because of it, but the reaction to it does. I loved my mother, but I couldn't honestly say that if I was able to, I would have wanted to be her caregiver. Too many buttons there to be pushed, if you will. My brother and sister were both there for her, and I would have been, but that's a matter of traditional family obligation for me, and each of them had their own reasons. They don't talk about it, and I've learned it isn't worth asking as it just causes issues to arise for all of us. So I and we allow sleeping dogs to mostly lie, and I am the only one left who is still a caregiver.

I am content in my role, and know positively that my wife loves me deeply. Hopefully my wife will be able to recover something resembling a decent mode of life in the not too distant future, and we will progress into mutual old age together. My brother is now retired and moved near my sister, in order to be around family as he ages. While not stated, we know he will also have family near should he become incapacitated. My sister continued working until this year, especially so as she had lost her vested interests in her retirement while being mom's caregiver. The hospital she worked for made her redundant in a sale to a different sort of care management corporation, she kept being offered lesser and lesser jobs because no one wanted to pay her what she was worth as a nurse of so many years experience, and well frankly, she also got tired of it all. She is now living with her kids in a mother's in law cottage, and finally has all the family she can possibly wish for, or not as she chooses. The same goes for my sister in law, who is surrounded by her family and husband as well. All four of us seniors survived my mother's declining years. Three were directly involved in her care, two had their lives radically changed as a result, and both of them have paid the price for the privilege and honor. Which once more gets us back to the beginning of this book, and its warning. Was the price worth it for them, yes, as far as they are concerned. If I should ever revise this book again, and they have both passed, perhaps I will detail the costs. But for now, if I were to do so, they would be very upset with me.

As for the third, my sister in law, well she lost our mother shortly after losing her own, and her sister. But she, notwithstanding the fact that she is one of the sweetest people one is likely to meet, was as affected by our mother's death as we all were. However, she also had and has one thing going for her which has kept her maintaining. Simply put, she has a truly deep and unwavering belief in a higher power, in her case, God. It is simple, unpretentious, but it has sustained her through her whole life. For myself, I frankly fought against religion for the first third of my life, but I have, if you will come to terms with God (on his terms), and my belief has kept me going through the worst of times, too. My sister and brother too, have their own beliefs, and while they prefer not to talk about them, I suppose their beliefs have helped them get to where they are now.

My second brother's death came out of the blue to our family, was sudden, and quick. My father's was in the hospital after several heart attacks. Now that was in the days when a bypass operation was relatively new, and very risky. However the option was offered. I was the youngest member of the family, and I was waiting for the responsible older ones to decide what to do. They had great difficulty, and finally asked my opinion. I asked the doctor is he would be able to climb stairs if the operation was a success. He said definitely not. Now my father's greatest pleasure was tinkering in his workshop, in the basement, one flight of steps down. His sanctuary was his office, one flight of steps upstairs. I knew that he would never really be happy without those two options, and so I was honest and said that unless he woke up and could make the decision himself, it would probably be best to let him go. He passed that night.

Was it the right decision, I don't know, but he passed on that night. Forty years later however, my remaining brother told me that he still couldn't forgive me for that decision. Okay, I was twenty-two years old at the time, and tried to guess what my father would have wanted. The operation was novel enough that he probably wouldn't have survived it. However, even my second brother told me shortly after Dad's death that he hated me for that decision (he got over that quickly). However, what the heck did my family want from me? I ventured an opinion and they jointly or severally could have decided otherwise. My mother, my eldest brother, my second brother and his wife, and finally my sister could have all spoken up and taken responsibility for the decision, but they left it with mine. Dad was okay with it, I believe, because I talked about it with him. I mean he was unconscious, but I believe he was in agreement none the less. And in the end, I believe God was glad to have him and later, my second brother and mother as well with him.

I decided to describe all of the above because I thought you should be privy to at least one specific death that did not involved years of caregiving and or deteriorating mental capacities. If you are keeping count, I was wrong in my choices to at least half the family, then, and because I was honest when it came to my relationship with my mother, the goat there, too. My relationship with God has kept me going however, and it will ultimately be his that I think will matter in the end. As I wrote earlier in this book, I personally see my departed loved ones all having a grand old time up there in heaven, and one day I will join them, hopefully after my wife's passing. She and I and them will then be together again, and sooner or later so will my remaining siblings. I think we will by that time all get along...

Whether or not you folks out there who read this believe in God or any other higher power is strictly up to you. It is my considered opinion however that if you do take up the gauntlet of being a caregiver, especially a twenty-four hour/ three hundred and sixty-five day a year one, you will need that belief to make it through to whatever finish line awaits. And personally, I think whether or not you believe in God, he believes in you.

So okay,

on

to

the

reference

section!

Wait a minute here. If you are buying the hard bound version of this book, then you will have to also get the hard bound version of the reference section, which is part two. It is over four hundred pages, ridiculously expensive, and ninety three plus percent of it will not be pertinent to you or the state in which you and your loved one reside. Please do us both a favor and pick up that section for <u>FREE</u> in the Kindle lending library, or just buy the whole thing at the reasonable price of 99 cents in its original Kindle version. Thank you.